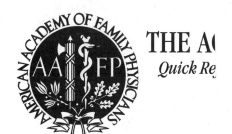

THE A(

Quick Re

Women's Health

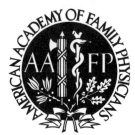

THE ACADEMY COLLECTION
Quick Reference Guides for Family Physicians

Women's Health

C. CAROLYN THIEDKE, MD
Assistant Professor of Family Medicine
Medical University of South Carolina
Charleston, South Carolina

JO ANN ROSENFELD, MD
Director of Women's Health
Franklin Square Family Practice Residency
Baltimore, Maryland

With

Rick D. Kellerman, MD
Professor and Chair of Family and
Community Medicine
University of Kansas at Wichita
Wichita, Kansas

Series Medical Editor
Richard Sadovsky, MD, MS
Associate Professor of Family Medicine
State University of New York Health Science Center
Brooklyn, New York

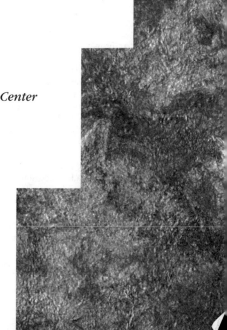

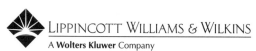

LIPPINCOTT WILLIAMS & WILKINS
A **Wolters Kluwer** Company
Philadelphia · Baltimore · New York · London
Buenos Aires · Hong Kong · Sydney · Tokyo

Acquisitions Editor: Richard Winters
Developmental Editor: Alexandra T. Anderson
Production Editor: Jeff Somers
Manufacturing Manager: Colin J. Warnock
Cover Designer: Jeane Norton
Compositor: Lippincott Williams & Wilkins Desktop Division
Printer: R. R. Donnelley, Crawfordsville

Library of Congress Cataloging-in-Publication Data
Thiedke, C. Carolyn
  Women's health / C. Carolyn Thiedke, Jo Ann Rosenfeld; with Rick D. Kellerman.
    p. cm.—(The Academy collection—quick reference guides for family physicians)
  Includes bibliographical references and index.
  ISBN 0-7817-2447-3 (alk. paper)
  1. Women—Health and hygiene.   I. Rosenfeld, Jo Ann.   II. Kellerman, Rick D.
III. Title.   IV. Series
RA778.T47 2000
613'.04244—dc21

                                                                00-025887

10 9 8 7 6 5 4 3 2 1

To my husband, Fred Thompson, and my children
John and Edward Thompson,
for the way they keep me grounded
in what's really important.

CCT

To Judy, my mother.

JAR

Contents

Acknowledgments ix

Preface xi

Series Introduction xiii

Chapter 1. Contraception *1*
            Jo Ann Rosenfeld

Chapter 2. Gynecologic Cancers *29*
            Jo Ann Rosenfeld and Rick Kellerman

Chapter 3. Breast Disease *45*
            Jo Ann Rosenfeld

Chapter 4. Menopause *59*
            C. Carolyn Thiedke

Chapter 5. Heart Disease *73*
            Jo Ann Rosenfeld

Chapter 6. Weight-Related Issues *85*
            C. Carolyn Thiedke

Chapter 7. Depression and Other Mood Disorders *103*
            C. Carolyn Thiedke

Chapter 8. Sexual Issues for Women *121*
            C. Carolyn Thiedke

Chapter 9. Osteoarthritis, Rheumatoid Arthritis, and
            Osteoporosis *135*
            Jo Ann Rosenfeld

Chapter 10. Fibromyalgia and Chronic Fatigue Syndrome *145*
            C. Carolyn Thiedke

Subject Index *157*

ACKNOWLEDGMENTS

Dr. Thiedke thanks Bill Simpson, M.D., her mentor, for his encouragement. She also thanks Erica Seastrunk and Joseph Greene for technical support, and Debbie Carson, Pharm.D., for her help with the section on medications used in menopause.

PREFACE

In the 20-year span of my professional career, I have been privileged to witness two waves in women's health care. The first came on the heels of the women's liberation movement, family-centered birth, and the ground-breaking book *Our Bodies, Ourselves*. It was a personal liberation that encouraged women to take control of their health, to explore their bodies, and to embrace their sexuality. In the physician's office women asked to be heard, to be taken seriously, and to be given control of health care decisions that affected them.

The second wave developed within the last decade and was a more public one. Inequities in funding for diseases that primarily affect women in most major research trials came to light. The outcry for fairness led to the creation of a division dedicated to women's health within most of the major governmental health agencies, including the National Institutes of Health, the Food and Drug Administration, the Centers for Disease Control, and the Department of Health and Human Services. The Women's Health Initiative, one of the largest prevention trials ever launched in the United States, began in 1991 with the hope that it would answer many of the tough questions facing women and their physicians today about hormone replacement, cardiovascular disease prevention, breast cancer, osteoporosis, and lifestyle changes.

When interest in women's health was at a peak in the early 1990s, many called for a new specialty in women's health. Although I was innervated by this interest in women's health, I believed that the creation of a new specialty was a bad idea. I feared that carving out a specialty in women's health would ultimately relegate these important issues to secondary status, but more importantly than that, I believed that the ideal practitioner for women's health already existed—the family physician.

I believe that family physicians, with their training in gynecology, behavioral science, preventive care, cardiovascular disease, and musculoskeletal disease, have the expertise to respond to all of women's health care needs. I also believe that most of my colleagues, both men and women, are empathic, caring individuals who have the communication skills that women value so highly in a doctor-patient interaction.

In the early days of the feminist movement, it seemed necessary to believe that women and men were basically the same, that only our socialization made us different. However, writers such as Carol Gilligan (*A Different Voice*) and Deborah Tannen (*You Just Don't Understand*) have shown that there are real differences in the communication styles of men and women. For physicians to work successfully with women patients, these differences must be appreciated.

In addition to the well-known fact that women see physicians much more frequently than men, studies have shown that women behave differently in the physician's office than men do. In general, women ask for more information and volunteer more information than men. Women more often express emotion and more often make statements that request collaboration with their physicians.

Surveys of women's preferences during visits with their doctors indicate a strong desire for an initial time to talk, a display of genuine concern through attentiveness, and a feeling that they are being treated as equals and are not being patronized. They want to have procedures explained to them, particularly those associated with a pelvic examination; they want their physicians to bring up sexual issues; and they want their physicians to talk to them when they are fully clothed. All of these skills are firmly entrenched in family practice training.

My coauthor, Dr. Joanne Rosenfeld, and I have attempted to produce a book that communicates a deep respect for women. We selected 10 top concerns, gynecologic and otherwise, that bring women to their physicians or that represent major health issues for women. We believe we have achieved the goal of this series: to produce books by practicing family physicians that wed current research with practical information in a format that is accessible. We hope we have woven advice into the book that will foster improved satisfaction with health care visits, not only for patients but for the physicians who care for them.

The 10-chapter format, of necessity, means that certain important topics could not be included. One topic encountered frequently, but without a section of its own, is the victimization of women through sexual abuse and domestic violence. These shadow issues often profoundly influence a doctor-patient interaction without the physician's awareness. We encourage physicians to maintain a high index of suspicion for abuse, particularly when meeting with challenging patients, and to include screening questions about abuse in their visits with women.

C. Carolyn Thiedke

SERIES INTRODUCTION

....

Family practice is a unique clinical specialty encompassing a philosophy of care rather than a modality of care provided to a specific segment of the population. This philosophy of providing longitudinal care for persons of all ages in the complete context of their physical, emotional, and social environments was modeled by general practitioners, the parents of our modern specialty. To provide this kind of care, the family physician needs a broad knowledge base, appropriate evaluation tools, effective interventions, and patient education.

The knowledge base needed by a family physician is extraordinarily large. The American Academy of Family Physicians and other organizations provide clinical education to practitioners through conferences and journals. Individual family physicians have written journal articles about specific clinical topics or have tried to cover the broad knowledge base of family medicine in a single volume. The former are helpful, but may cover only a narrow segment of medicine, while the latter may not provide the depth needed to be useful in actual patient care.

The Academy Collection: Quick Reference Guides for Family Physicians is a series of books designed to assist family physicians with the broad knowledge base unique to our specialty. The books in this series have all been written by practicing family physicians who have special interest in the topics, and the chapters have been formatted to provide easy access to information needed at varying stages in the physician-patient encounter. Each volume is unique because each author has personalized the volume and provided a unique family physician perspective.

This series is not meant to be a final reference for the family physician who seeks a comprehensive text. The series also does not cover every topic that may be encountered by the family physician. The series does offer, in a depth deemed appropriate by the authors, the information needed by the physician to handle most patient encounters. The series also provides information to make patient care a combined doctor-patient effort. Specific patient education materials have been included where appropriate. Readers can contact the American Academy of Family Physicians Foundation for other resources.

The topics selected for *The Academy Collection* were chosen based on what family physicians said they needed. The first group of books covers office procedures, conditions of aging, and some of the most challenging diagnoses seen in family practice. Future books in the series will address musculoskeletal problems, environmental medicine, children's health, gastrointestinal problems, and women's health issues.

I welcome your comments. Please contact me at the American Academy of Family Physicians with your suggestions (Rick Sadovsky, MD, Series Editor, *The Academy Collection*, c/o AAFP, 11400 Tomahawk Creek Parkway, Leawood, KS 66211-2672; e-mail: academycollection@aafp.org). This collection is meant to be useful to you and your patients.

Richard Sadovsky, M.D., M.S.
Series Editor

CHAPTER 1

Contraception

Jo Ann Rosenfeld

Contraception provides a sexually active woman with the ability to prevent conception. The choice of contraception must take into consideration the woman's lifestyle, preferences, concerns, and health problems. Physicians and women must work cooperatively to help find the best method for the woman.

FACTORS IN CHOICE OF CONTRACEPTION

Many factors must be considered when a physician helps a woman choose a method of contraception. Working collaboratively, the physician and woman can evaluate the options and make the best choice. This discussion should be interactive and sensitive to the woman's needs and beliefs about contraception (Table 1.1).

T ABLE 1.1. Classification of methods

1. Lack-of-contact methods
   a. Abstinence
   b. Periodic abstinence or rhythm
   c. Natural family planning (NFP)
   d. Coitus interruptus (withdrawal)
2. Barrier methods
   a. Male condoms
   b. Female condoms
   c. Diaphragms
   d. Caps
   e. Spermicides
3. Hormonal methods
   a. Emergency contraception or the morning-after pill
   b. Oral contraceptives (OCPs) of the following kinds
      (1) Regular (fixed combinations of estrogen and progesterone)
      (2) Triphasic (fixed concentration of estrogen with changing concentrations of progesterone)
      (3) Second generation (use of desogestrel or gestodene for the progesterone)
      (4) Third generation (use of norgestrel or levonorgestril for the progesterone)
      (5) Progestin-only pills
      (6) New low-dose estrogen or changing-dose estrogen pills
   c. Implantable rods of hormones
   d. Injectable contraception (depo-medroxyprogesterone [DMP] Depo-Provera)
   e. Intrauterine device
4. Sterilization

T ABLE 1.2.   Contraceptive-method choices depending on desire for future fertility

Good Choice for Immediate Return to Fertility on Cessation	Intermediate Time Needed for Return to Fertility	Inappropriate Use if Future Fertility Wanted
Abstinence, rhythm, NFP, CI	OCPs (6–12 months)	IUDs
Barrier methods	DMP (12–24 months)	Sterilization
Emergency contraception	Norplant (must be removed)	

Abbreviations: CI, coitus interruptus; DMP, depomedroxyprogesterone; IUD, intrauterine device; NFP, natural family planning; OCPs, oral contraceptive pills.

Personal and Medical History

Desire for Future Fertility

A woman needs to ask herself if she wants to become pregnant and, if so, when (Table 1.2). Younger women, single women, and those who know they want more children in the near future should use an easily reversible form of contraception. Women who are certain they have finished childbearing may desire a permanent form of contraception.

- **Immediate reversibility.** Lack-of-contact methods (such as abstinence, natural family planning, and so on), barrier methods, and emergency contraception (EC) are immediately reversible.
- **Intermediate reversibility.** With oral contraceptive pills (OCPs), return to fertility may take 6 to 12 months. With depo-medroxyprogesterone (DMP), the return to fertility may take as long as 24 months. After cessation, it is common for amenorrhea or anovulatory cycles to last from 6 to 12 months. For levonorgestrel implants (Norplant), return to ovulation is the same as that with OCPs (Fig. 1.1).
- **Permanent sterilization.** Sterilization must be considered permanent, although both tubal ligation (TL) and vasectomy can be surgically reversed. Removal of intrauterine devices (IUDs) imparts return to fertility immediately, but sterility is a risk.

Menstrual History Problems

Menorrhagia or Dysmenorrhea   If a woman has a history of menorrhagia or dysmenorrhea, OCPs may be a very good choice because they decrease the flow and pain of menstrual periods. OCPs also improve the regularity of menstrual periods (Table 1.3). On the other hand, with DMP and Norplant there is significant breakthrough bleeding (BTB), especially in the first few

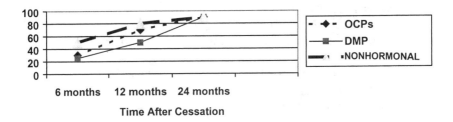

FIGURE 1.1.   Cumulative contraception rates after cessation of contraception. OCP, oral contraceptive pills; DMP, depo-medroxyprogesterone.

TABLE 1.3. Types of oral contraceptives

Oral Contraceptives	Type of Pill	Amount and Type of Estrogen	Amount and Type of Progesterone	Comments
First-generation noncyclic				
Ortho Novum 1/50, Norinyl 1/50	Regular—constant	50 μg mestranol	1 mg norethindrone	High-dose estrogen, standard pill, often used for BTB
Ortho Novum 1/35, Norinyl 1/35	Regular—constant	35 μg EE	1 mg norethindrone	Standard pill
Ovral	Constant	50 μg EE	0.5 mg norgestrel	Constant doses of high-dose androgenic progestin and estrogen used for women with problems of BTB. High chance of acne
Lo-Ovral, Nordette, Levlen	Constant, low estrogen	30 μg EE	0.15–0.3 mg norgestrel	Constant doses of low-dose estrogen but with progestins of high androgenic power. To help women with BTB. High chance of acne
First Generation—Cyclic Pills				
Ortho-Novum 7/7/7 Tri-Norinyl	Constant estrogen dose, variable progestin / Cyclic	35 μg EE	Varying amounts of norethindrone throughout the month, none more than 1 mg per day	Standard starting pill today
Triphasil, Tri-Levlen	Cyclic	30–40 μg EE	0.05–0.125 mg of levonorgestrel	
Second Generation	Constant estrogen doses, new progestins—some cyclic			
Ortho-Cept	Second generation—constant doses	30 μg EE	0.15 mg desogestrel	Less BTB
Ortho Tri-cyclen, Ortho-Cyclen	Cyclic—second generation	35 μg EE	0.18–0.25 mg norgestimate	Less BTB
Low-Estrogen Pills				
Estrostep	Cyclic changing of estrogen	5 days of 20 μg, 7 days of 30 μg, 9 days of 35 μg EE	1 mg norethindrone	Seven tablets of ferrous fumarate 75 mg instead of sugar pills
Third-Generation Combination				
Alesse, Levlen	Low-dose estrogen but constant	20–30 mcg EE	0.1–0.15 mg levonorgestrel	Less BTB
Progestin-Only	Progestin-only			
Ovrette		None	0.075 mg norgestrel	Less estrogen side effects. Use in women with estrogen problems
Micronor		None	0.35 mg norethindrone	

Abbreviations: BTB, breakthrough bleeding; EE, ethinyl estradiol.

months. This does improve in time. With 6 to 12 months of use, women taking DMP usually become amenorrheic, and those taking Norplant have regular cycles.

IUDs and TL are known to cause heavier menstrual periods and should be avoided in women with menorrhagia.

Oligomenorrhea Women with oligomenorrhea may have regular periods with OCPs and should avoid DMP.

Abnormal Pap Tests

Women with a history of abnormal Pap tests may need to avoid hormonal contraceptives, especially until the abnormality is evaluated and treated. Women who have or have had cervical cancer should avoid hormonal contraceptives. There is an increased risk of cervical cancer in women who use OCPs, and the risk increases the longer the woman uses OCPs. Women who currently use combination OCPs have a 10.9 times greater risk of precancerous lesions (squamous intraepithelial neoplasia).

Gynecologic Abnormalities

Women with structural gynecologic abnormalities may not do well with barrier contraceptives, especially diaphragms, cervical caps, and female condoms, because they may not fit. Whether they can take hormonal contraceptives depends on the abnormality.

Women with structural abnormalities of the cervix or uterus may do well with OCPs, Norplant, or DMP. An IUD would be difficult to place in a woman with a double cervix or uterus and might not work in the other horn or uterus.

Medical Problems

Many medical problems can require a change in choice of contraception. Hormonal contraceptives may be contraindicated, or should only be taken with caution and close medical observation in women with some medical diseases or conditions (Tables 1.4, 1.5, and 1.6). Recently, however, women with conditions that once were considered absolute or relative contraindications for hormonal contraception have been using OCPs or the progestin-only OCPs. One reason that some conditions are no longer considered absolute contraindications is that all forms of contraception have lower morbidity and mortality rates than those with pregnancy, at least until 45 years of age. Only smokers who are more than 35 years of age and take OCPs (especially those beyond the age of 45) have higher morbidity and mortality rates than pregnant

T ABLE 1.4.   Medical conditions that are absolute contraindications to OCPs

Smoker over age 35
Active and symptomatic gallstones
Unexplained vaginal bleeding
Pregnancy
Unexplained liver function tests or liver mass
History of thromboembolism—deep venous thrombosis, pulmonary embolism, cerebrovascular accident
Hyperlipidemia (triglycerides >750 mg/dL)
Lupus erythematosus
Estrogen- or progesterone-dependent cancer—ovarian, cervical, endometrial

TABLE 1.5. Medical conditions that are relative contraindications to OCPs

Condition	OCPs may be used if condition:
History of gallstones	Is asymptomatic
Diabetes	Is not worsened by OCPs
Hypertension	Is not worsened by OCPs
Hepatitis	Is stable and controlled
Hyperlipidemia	Is triglycerides < 750 mg/dL and not worsened by OCPs
Migraine headaches	Is not worsened by OCPs

Abbreviation: OCPs, oral contraceptive pills.

women of the same age. Thus a diabetic or hypertensive woman whose disease is well controlled and who is taking an OCP has a lower risk of illness and death than if she were to become pregnant.

Several medical conditions can sometimes be worsened by estrogen-containing OCPs. However, these OCPs can be used if the woman and her physician closely follow her condition (Table 1.4). Alternatively, progestin-only OCPs, Norplant, or DMP can be used in some situations (Tables 1.5 and 1.6).

Women with mild forms of hyperlipidemia can use progestin-only OCPs. Combination OCPs can be used in women who do not have vascular disease, do not smoke, and have well-controlled lipid levels.

Women who have bleeding disorders may do better on OCPs because they decrease the amount of menstrual blood. If headaches are not worsened by OCPs, women can continue them. Women with seizure disorders can take OCPs, but medication levels may need to be monitored (see later). Women with psychiatric disturbances, including schizophrenia, manic-depressive disorders, and depression, often do better on a predictable contraceptive provided by OCPs, Norplant, or DMP. These women may do even better on DMP because it requires no daily involvement. However, medication levels may need close follow-up.

Barrier methods are not contraindicated in any medical condition. However, women with vaginal or cervical infections or rashes should have these treated before barrier methods or spermicides are used.

Medication Use

Barrier methods, contact methods, or sterilization are not affected by medications. Many medications, especially hormonal medication, may make menstrual periods irregular and create difficulty for women using rhythm or natural family planning (NFP). A number of medications can affect OCPs significantly or interfere with their metabolism (Table 1.7).

Cost

Methods vary by cost per use and per year. Cost has not been shown to inhibit use of contraception (Table 1.8).

Availability

Ease of availability may make a difference to some couples as they assess methods. Coitus interruptus (CI), although not reliable, is always readily available. Condoms and spermicides are readily available over the counter. Use of the rhythm method, or NFP,

T ABLE 1.6. Use of OCPs in medical conditions

Medical Condition	Can Use Combination OCPs	Can Use Progestin-Only OCPs	Comments
Benign breast disease	Yes	Yes	Benign breast disease, especially fibrocystic disease, can be improved by OCP use.
Depression	Yes	Yes	OCPs have no proven effect on mood.
Diabetes mellitus	Yes	Yes	OCPs can be used by women with type I or II diabetes mellitus, who are younger than age 35, are otherwise healthy, and do not smoke or have vascular complications.
Gestational diabetes	Yes	Yes	No contraindication.
Gallbladder disease	Conditional	Yes	OCP use may hasten an attack in a woman with stones or a history of stones.
Congenital or valvular heart disease	Conditional	Yes	Only contraindicated if the woman has marginal reserves or a condition that predisposes to thrombosis.
Hemorrhagic disorders	Yes	Yes	Even women with anticoagulants can use OCPs. They may decrease bleeding and prevent hemorrhagic corpus luteum.
Hepatic disease	Conditional	Conditional	If the cause of the liver damage is known and the liver function tests have returned to normal.
Hyperlipidemia	Conditional	Conditional	If the woman has uncontrolled hypercholesterolemia or hypertriglyceridemia or vascular disease or smokes, OCPs should not be used. In women with hypertriglyceridemia, if tricylerides can be controlled (750 mg/dL), OCPs, especially progestin-only OCPs, can be tried.
Hypertension	Yes	Yes	If hypertension is controlled, OCPs can be used with close follow-up.
Pregnancy-induced hypertension	Conditional	Conditional	Once hypertension is controlled, OCPs can be used.
Migraine headaches	Conditional	Yes	Low-dose estrogen OCPs can be tried in women without neurologic symptoms. However, if headaches increase, OCPs must be stopped.

continued

TABLE 1.6 *continued.* Use of OCPs in medical conditions

Medical Condition	Can Use Combination OCPs	Can Use Progestin-Only OCPs	Comments
Mitral valve prolapse	Conditional	Yes	OCPs can be used in asymptomatic nonsmoking women. Women with atrial fibrillation or migraine headaches should only use progestin-only OCPs.
Obesity	Yes	Yes	
Seizure disorders	Yes	Yes	OCPs do not affect seizure threshold. However, they can affect metabolism of anticonvulsants, and anticonvulsants can inactivate OCPs; close follow-up is essential.
Sickle cell disease	Yes	Yes	
Smoking	No after age 35	Yes	In women older than age 35 who smoke and take OCPs the mortality rate is higher than in individuals who do not take OCPs. An ex-smoker can be considered a nonsmoker.
SLE	No	?	Estrogen-containing OCPs can worsen SLE.
Ulcerative colitis	Yes	Yes	OCPs are absorbed in the small bowel, not the colon.

Abbreviations: OCPs, oral contraceptive pills; SLE, systemic lupus erythematosus.

requires knowledge of when in the month the woman is fertile and avoiding intercourse at that time. This method is available to most women, although proper use requires access to a coach/teacher and strong commitment. Hormonal methods, diaphragms, and cervical caps can require a visit to a physician but should be readily available. Regular follow-up visits are needed to make these methods efficient because a new size or prescription may be needed. IUD, Norplant, and sterilization initially require a visit and procedure, but then they are effective for a long time (permanently, in the case of sterilization).

Sexual Experiences
How couples experience sexual relations may affect the contraceptive method they use. Some methods can be viewed as an inconvenience or as part of foreplay (e.g., putting in a diaphragm or putting on a condom). Some couples prefer that contraception be physically removed from the sexual experience and thus may choose hormonal methods or sterilization. CI may be totally unacceptable to some couples and decreases the woman's sexual satisfaction unless nonpenetration methods of producing orgasm are also used. There is some evidence that women who are not happy with sexual intimacy are less likely to use contraceptives effectively.

T ABLE 1.7.   Interaction between oral contraceptives and some medications

Drugs Whose Activity May Be Reduced by OCPs
Acetaminophen
Benzodiazepines—lorazepam, oxazepam, temazepam (those renally excreted)
Water-soluble vitamins

Drugs Whose Levels and Activity May Be Increased by OCPs
Benzodiazepines—alprazolam, chlordiazepoxide, clorazepate, diazepam, flurazepam, triazolam
Beta-blockers
Caffeine
Clofibrate
Corticosteroids
Salicylates
Theophylline
Tricyclic antidepressants
Fat-soluble vitamins

Drugs That May Reduce OCP Efficacy, Causing Ovulation
Antifungal drugs
Antibiotics
  Tetracycline, doxycycline
  Ampicillin
  Antituberculosis drugs, including rifampin
Anticonvulsants
Sedatives

Drugs That May Increase Levels of Estrogen or Enhance OCP Efficacy
Vitamin C

Abbreviation: OCPs, oral contraceptive pills.

Orderliness of Life

How often, where, and when a woman expects or plans sexual intercourse, or if she can plan sexual intercourse, may affect what method is most acceptable to her. Certainly, couples cannot use the rhythm method unless they can plan when they are having sex. Teenagers or college-age women may not know when or where sex may occur and thus must either plan ahead by using hormonal contraception or having condoms or other barrier methods on hand when they may be needed. Diaphragms left at home do not work. Married couples who usually have sexual intercourse in the same place and can plan their relations may not need the ease of availability of condoms, and diaphragms may work well for them. If a woman works different shifts or travels, it may be difficult for her to take OCPs with her so that she can take them at approximately the same time every day. Norplant or DMP may be a better choice.

Occupation

Although no employer can forbid a woman an occupation because of risk to unborn fetuses, some professions involve toxic or infectious exposures that may make it inad-

T ABLE 1.8. Financial costs of contraception

Method	Cost/Sexual Intercourse	Cost/Year*
Abstinence	No cost	None
Rhythm	No cost	None
NFP	Variable—cost for training, one-time fee	$10, $100–$300 total
Coitus interruptus	No cost	None
Spermicides	$1–3	$150–$450
Condoms, male	Variable—latex, from free to $3/condom; polyurethane, more expensive	0 to $150–$200 or more
Condoms, female	$3	$450
Diaphragm	Doctor's visit, approximately $25–$30/ diaphragm plus spermicides	$250–$550
IUD	$150–$250 plus insertion by physician approximately $350–$500 total	$80
Depo-Provera	$45/injection plus one doctor's visit	$120
Norplant	$500 insertion, $250–$350 removal	$100
OCPs	$25–$30/month plus doctor's visit	$475
EC	$5–$30 plus possible doctor's visit	Variable
Sterilization, male	Approximately $1,200	$40†
Sterilization, female	Approximately $1,200–$2,500	$40–$80†

Abbreviations: EC, emergency contraception; IUD, intrauterine device; NFP, natural family planning; OCPs, oral contraceptive pills.

*Assuming 30-year fertility and sexual intercourse approximately three times a week.

†Dependent on the number of years used.

visable for a woman to become pregnant (Table 1.9). If a woman may be exposed to teratogenic toxins, she may want a very effective contraceptive that has few to no failures, no matter what side effects. A woman anesthetist, anesthesiologist, or chemist may choose DMP, Norplant, OCPs, IUDs, or sterilization. Similarly, a nurse or physician who may be exposed to blood products that are infected with the AIDS virus may also want very effective contraception.

T ABLE 1.9. Occupations in which there may be a significant hazard to getting pregnant or being pregnant

Chemical exposures
  Anesthesia: nurses, anesthetists, anesthesiologists
  Toxins: chemical workers, dyes, plastics
Radiation exposures
Infectious exposures (including exposure to AIDS, rubella, meningococcemia, hepatitis, cytomegalovirus, and others): nurses, health care workers, day care workers

Side Effects and Women's Concerns

For failure rates and side effects of some forms of emergency contraception see Fig. 1.2.

Breakthrough Bleeding

Some women find BTB unacceptable, especially if it impedes their daily activities or sexual life. For these women, OCPs with little BTB (second- and third-generation pills, Ovral, Lo/Ovral, or cyclic pills) may be the best choice. The newer second- or third-generation pills have a BTB rate of only 7% in the first 3 months and less than 3% by 6 months. Women who are concerned about BTB may not tolerate the BTB of the first 3 to 6 months of DMP or Norplant use.

Fear of Cancer

Fear of cancer may keep some women from using certain methods, especially hormonal methods. Despite evidence and physician information, many women believe pills and contraception are far less effective and far less safe than evidence has shown. These beliefs are affected by the woman's culture and must be discussed as part of a complete discussion of contraception.

Although having an estrogen-dependent cancer would be a contraindication for many forms of hormonal contraception, these methods do not increase the risk of this type of cancer in most populations. Information and reassurance may help women and couples accept and feel comfortable with these methods despite their fears. It may be helpful to share the following information with women:

1. **Barrier methods.** The cervical cap has been associated with an increase in incidence of abnormal Pap tests, but not an increase in cervical cancer.
2. **Hormonal methods.** Although some women fear an increased risk of cancer, hormonal contraception may actually decrease the risk of ovarian and endometrial cancers. Use of OCPs has been associated with a definite decrease in the incidence in cancers of the endometrium and may decrease the risk of epithelial ovarian cancer. Use of OCPs does not increase the risk of cervical dysplasia. Use of OCPs lowers the incidence of benign breast disease. A case-controlled study between 1983 and 1988 showed that, compared with no use, using combination OCPs for 12 years or more was associated with a modest increase in the risk of breast cancer.

Evidence suggests that progestin-only pills, DMP, and Norplant do not increase the risk of breast cancer, invasive adenocarcinomas of the cervix, or squamous cer-

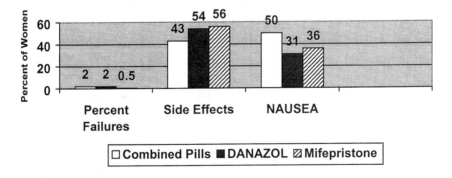

FIGURE 1.2. Failure rates and side effects of some forms of emergency contraception. (These medications are not FDA approved for this indication.)

vical cancer. Use of progestin-only pills created a relative risk of 1.1 for breast cancer in one study of 900 women. DMP may be protective against the development of leiomyomas of the uterus.

Fear of DVTs

Women who use OCPs definitely have an increased risk of all thromboembolic disease. The risk of deep venous thrombosis (DVT) and thromboembolic disease is related to the dose of estrogen. When doses of estrogen decreased to 35 µg or less of ethinyl estradiol, the rates of DVT decreased, although the risk is still two times greater than that for women who do not take OCPs. However, stroke and death from thromboembolism are very rare and no statistically significant increase in risk could be attributed to OCPs. Whereas the risk of DVT with OCPs with less than 50 µg of ethinyl estradiol is 15 per 100,000 individuals, the risk of DVT with pregnancy is 60 per 100,000.

Strokes

No method of contraception increases the risk of stroke. Even combination OCPs, with less than 50 µg of estrogen, do not increase the risk of strokes, either ischemic or hemorrhagic. OCPs with 50 µg of estrogen increased blood pressure to hypertensive levels (a risk factor for stroke) in approximately 5% of users, in a study of more than 68,000 women. The age-adjusted rate of hypertension in women who used OCPs was 1.5 in current users and 1.1 in past users.

Heart Attacks

OCPs decrease the risk of myocardial infarction.

Osteoporosis

Combination OCPs appear likely to increase bone density. There is some evidence that long-term use of Depo-Provera may decrease bone density, but its effect is not well defined.

METHODS

Lack-of-Contact Methods

Opinions of various contraceptive methods from women in the United States, the Netherlands, and Canada are shown in Fig. 1.3.

Abstinence

- **Efficacy.** Abstinence is an excellent method of contraception with an unfortunate high rate of human failure, giving it a 50% failure rate (Fig. 1.4).
- **Indications.** It is a good method for teenagers and absolutely protective against pregnancy and STDs. It costs nothing and is easily available.
- **Contraindications.** It is difficult to achieve consistently.
- **STD protection.** Complete if used properly.

Coitus Interruptus

- **Efficacy.** The success rate of CI depends on the couple. Teenagers have more trouble; with typical use the efficacy rate is 81%. The rate may be much lower in some populations. In couples who use this method perfectly, efficacy rates of 96% have been achieved.
- **Indications.** This may be best in monogamous or mature couples who can discuss their sexual experiences and learn each other's cues and can accept the risk of pregnancy. In addition, this is good for those who dislike hormonal contraception.

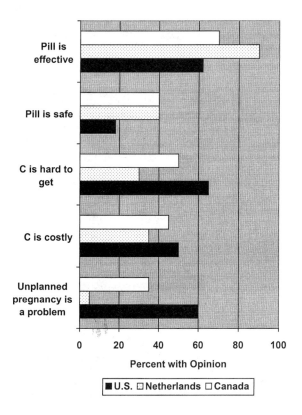

FIGURE 1.3. Opinions of contraception. C, contraception.

Achieving effective CI may be a good way for a couple to establish effective communication skills.
- **Cost/availability.** This is free and readily available.
- **Contraindications.** If a woman must not get pregnant, this is a poor choice. Unless stimulation other than with penetration is used, a woman's satisfaction and orgasms may be adversely affected.
- **STD protection.** Variable.

Rhythm—Periodic Abstinence

Rhythm, or periodic abstinence, depends on knowing when a woman is fertile based on dating menstrual periods and restricting intercourse to the "safe" period in the menstrual cycle. Sperm can remain active and capable of fertilizing an egg from 2 to 4 days after sex. The couple abstains from sexual relations 2 to 4 days before and after ovulation (that date should be 14 days before her next menstrual period). If she has regular periods every 28 days, the couple would abstain from day 11 or 12 to day 16 or 17 of her menstrual period. If she has 31 to 33 days in her menstrual cycle (a bit irregular), the couple must abstain from day 14 to day 21.

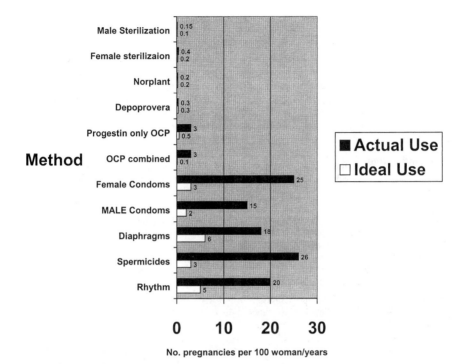

FIGURE 1.4. Failure rates of contraceptive methods. (Data from the Alan Guttmacher Institute, 1995.) OCP, oral contraceptive pills.

- **Efficacy.** In women with regular menstrual periods, this method can reach 91% efficacy. In women with irregular menstrual periods, an efficacy rate of 81% is more typical.
- **Indications.** Members of certain religious groups who do not desire an active contraceptive use this method. Women with regular menstrual periods have better results.
- **Cost/availability.** This is free. It is readily available, but sexual relations must be avoided from 4 to 8 days per month.
- **Contraindications.** Women with irregular periods, teenagers, and older women near menopause do poorly with this method.
- **STD protection.** None.

Natural Family Planning

Natural family planning (NFP) is a very well-established course of using rhythm and adding to it measurement of basal body temperatures and cervical mucus production to more accurately pinpoint the days before and after ovulation.

- **Efficacy.** With typical use the efficacy is 85%; with perfect use it is 98%.
- **Indications.** Because of the investment in time and commitment required, well-established couples may do better with it. Couples who do not wish to use hormones or active methods of contraception for religious purposes may prefer NFP.

- **Cost/availability.** An initial outlay of $200 to $400 is needed to enroll in the course; some catholic hospitals may offer free courses. No further cost is incurred. Once the course is taken, availability is good.
- **Contraindications.** Teenagers or singles are poor candidates. This method takes commitment and an almost compulsive continual determination of ovulation periods. Women with irregular menstrual bleeding or unexplained vaginal bleeding or discharge might have difficulty determining their cervical mucus periods and thus have trouble with this method. Women with irregular periods may be unable to determine their day of ovulation by basal body temperature measurement.
- **STD protection.** None.

Barrier Methods

Although barrier methods are very effective, they have to be used consistently. Even so, they occasionally fail. Of the 10 million women who use barrier contraception, approximately one-third report not using their method every time. One barrier method not discussed here is the contraceptive sponge. The manufacturer of the sponge applied to the U.S. FDA in January 2000 and is waiting to reintroduce the sponge to the U.S. market.

Gels, Creams, Suppositories

A wide variety of gels, creams, and suppositories are available with a variety of viscosities, ease of cleaning, smells, tastes, and ability to effervesce. Spermicides must be inserted before sexual intercourse and reapplied before subsequent intercourse. The woman cannot douche for 8 hours after sex.

- **Efficacy.** Between 79% and 97%.
- **Indications.** Women and couples who want an inexpensive method that does not require a visit with a health care provider and who do not want hormone side effects may appreciate spermicides. Use of a condom or diaphragm will increase the efficacy and considerably decrease the risk of STDs.
- **Cost/availability.** Cost is approximately $10 to $15 per tube of 8 to 10 applications, or about $1 to $2 per use. These products are easily obtainable at most grocery stores and pharmacies without a prescription.
- **Contraindications.** Women who become irritated with use of certain spermicides should avoid them. Irritative vaginitis is a possible complication. These methods can be messy.
- **STD protection.** Spermicides do provide some protection against AIDS, gonorrhea, syphilis, and chlamydia.

Male Condoms

Rubber condoms have been available since 1830 and have been made with good quality controls since the 1920s. Originally used for prophylaxis against STDs, contraception was a by-product. Use has increased significantly since the HIV/AIDS epidemic has targeted use of condoms to prevent HIV transmission. The proportion of women using condoms increased from 15% to 20% among all women, from 20% to 30% among never-married women, and from 33% to 37% among adolescents. More than one-third of teenage women using contraceptives choose condoms as their primary method. Condom use is lower among older women and married women .

- **Efficacy.** The efficacy ranges from 84% to 97%. Breakage occurs in approximately 1 in 100 uses. Condoms are excellent for prevention of STDs and AIDS and pregnancy. They are spontaneous and have no hormone effects. They are a good choice for new couples. They may be used in foreplay.
- **Cost/availability.** Cost ranges from free to $3 per condom. They can be bought without a physician's prescription at any drug or grocery store, or from dispensers in bathrooms.

- **Contraindications.** Many couples dislike the decrease in sensation and pleasure attributed to condoms. An allergy to latex would be a contraindication to normal condom use, but polyurethane condoms are now available.
- **STD protection.** Male condoms provide excellent STD and HIV/AIDS protection. When condoms are consistently used during heterosexual intercourse by couples with one member who is HIV-positive, transmission of HIV is greatly reduced.

Female Condoms

Only one company currently makes a female condom (the Reality condom), which makes availability more of an issue with female condoms. Less than 1% of women who use contraceptives use the female condom.
- **Efficacy.** Efficacy ranges from a low of 75% to 90%.
- **Indications.** Women who want to control their method and do not want hormonal side effects or a physician's visit may use female condoms. Women whose partners do not use male condoms and who want STD protection may desire this method.
- **Cost/availability.** Reality condoms cost $24 for eight condoms. Availability is difficult. Allergies to latex are a contraindication.
- **STD protection.** Unless the female condom slips out of place or is torn, it should provide protection as well as the male condom. However, there are no long-term data on whether the female condom prevents transmission of STDs. There is some evidence that African women whose husbands are HIV-positive and who use female condoms along with male condoms have a lower transmission rate.

Diaphragms

Diaphragms are a good method for committed women who have predictable sexual relationships. They must be used with spermicides and must be left in place for 8 hours after use. The longer women use them as a method, the better they work. They are not suction cups, do move with sex, and work by allowing more effective application of spermicide to the cervix.
- **Efficacy.** The efficacy of diaphragms ranges from 82% to 94%. They are less effective in women younger than 30 years of age and in women who have sex more than four times a week.
- **Indications.** Women who do not want hormonal effects or who have intermittent well-planned sexual intercourse will do well with diaphragms. Teenagers usually do not choose this method. Some couples use placement of a diaphragm as foreplay.
- **Cost/availability.** A diaphragm costs approximately $25 and lasts 1 year. A yearly visit to the physician for sizing and tests will most likely be needed. Diaphragms should be replaced after 1 year and must be used with spermicides, which adds a cost of $1 to $2 per sexual intercourse. Diaphragms must be refitted after a pregnancy or a weight gain or loss of 20 pounds. There are four types of diaphragms: arcing, coil, flat, and wide seal.
- **Contraindications.** Diaphragms have been associated with increased risk and incidence of urinary tract infections (UTI) and vaginal candidiasis, and should be avoided in women with these problems. They are not associated with cervical cytologic abnormalities. The continuation rate of diaphragms is only 35% for the first year of use.
- **STD protection.** With use of spermicides, diaphragms provide moderate protection against STDs.

Cervical Caps

In the United States, one company (Cervical Cap, Limited) is the sole distributor of the Prentif Cavity Rim Cervical Cap (made by Lamberts of London). Approximately 20% of women who request it cannot be fitted for the cap. The cervical cap provides contraceptive protection for 48 hours no matter how many times sexual intercourse occurs. It is not necessary to add additional spermicide each time.

- **Efficacy.** Efficacy ranges from 82% for usual use to 91% for nulliparous women and 74% for parous women.
- **Indications.** The cervical cap is indicated for women who understand their anatomy, have the anatomic ability to be sized and wear the cap, and can place it efficiently. Women must have the commitment to use it consistently.
- **Cost/availability.** The cost of a cervical cap is about $30 to $40. It should be replaced at least annually.
- **Contraindications.** Allergy to latex or abnormal gynecologic anatomy would be absolute contraindications. There is some evidence that cervical caps are associated with cervical abnormalities. Women with cervical Pap test abnormalities should use another form of contraception.
- **STDs.** Protects against many STDs, including HIV/AIDS.

Hormonal Methods
Emergency Contraception
Emergency contraception (EC), or the "morning-after pill," is used widely in Europe and is gaining popularity in the United States (Table 1.10). Used for failure of contraception (condom breakage) or failure to use contraception, it is an effective one-time method to prevent conception. Its mode of action was initially thought to be prevention of implantation, but evidence suggests that it also prevents conception. When an individual needs EC, an opportunity is created for counseling about long-term contraception.

There are now prescription packs of EC called Preven and Plan B. Preven has four pills (each containing ethinyl estradiol and levonorgestrel) and a pregnancy test. Plan B comes as a package of 2 pills. They cost approximately $23. There are other methods of EC, using various OCPs. With these the woman must take two doses, the first within 72 hours of coitus. The earlier she takes the pill, the more effective it is. Side

T ABLE 1.10. Emergency contraception

Brand	Pills per Dose	EE per Dose (μg)	Levonorgestrel per Dose (μg)†
Ovral	2 white pills*	100	0.50
Alesse	5 pink pills*	100	0.50
Levlen	4 light orange pills*	120	0.60
Lo/Ovral	4 white pills*	120	0.60
Triphasil	4 yellow pills*	120	0.50
Tri-Levlen	4 yellow pills*	120	0.50
Danazol**	800 mg (One tablet PO)		
Mifepristone,***	600 mg (One tablet PO)		
Preven	2 pills*	0.10 mg	0.50 mg
Plan B	1 pill*	0.75 mg	

Abbreviation: EE, ethinyl estradiol.

*The treatment regimen is one dose within 72 hours but as soon as possible after unprotected intercourse, and another dose 12 hours later. If nausea occurs and the woman vomits either dose, she should take them again after an antiemetic.

**Not FDA approved for this indication.

***Not available in the U.S.

†Norgestrel contains equal amounts of two isomers, of which only levonorgestrel is bioavailable.

effects include nausea and vomiting and breast tenderness, although Plan B causes less nausea. If the woman vomits her medication, she must take it again as soon as possible, perhaps after an antiemetic. Although it is not currently available in the United States, RU-486 (mifepristone) is a very effective method of EC and requires only one pill.

- **Efficacy.** Used appropriately, EC is 98% effective in preventing pregnancy.
- **Indications.** EC is indicated in contraception failure of method or intention.
- **Cost/availability.** The medication costs $5 to $25. A provider visit is necessary, however.
- **Contraindications.** Allergy to the ingredients or religious objections to possible prevention of implantation.
- **STDs.** No protection against STDs.

Combination Oral Contraceptives

Birth control pills (BCP) originally used high doses of estrogen; new OCPs use relatively lower doses, which decrease side effects while continuing high efficacy in preventing pregnancies. Many are available (Table 1.3). The pill is the most widely used method by women in their 20s. More than 1 million women in their teens, approximately 44%, use OCPs. Yet 1 million pregnancies a year occur because of imperfect use of OCPs.

Women have many fears about side effects and safety with OCPs. Although more than three-fourths of women in the United States have used OCPs sometime during their child-bearing years, fewer than one in five consider them safe. Despite evidence that OCPs decrease the risk of ovarian and endometrial cancer and only slightly increase (relative risk, 1.1) the risk of breast cancer, many women do not feel comfortable using them. Side effects such as BTB, breast changes, hair changes, weight gain, and headaches, whether proven or perceived, also decrease their use and acceptability. Newer second- and third-generation OCPs decrease the incidence of BTB significantly and the progestin-related side effects.

- **Efficacy.** Combination OCPs are incredibly effective: from 99.9% effective with ideal use to 94% with average use. Smoking cigarettes may decrease their effectiveness. Women who forget to take their pills should have a back-up contraceptive method, such as a barrier method.
- **Indications.** OCPs provide many benefits besides efficacious contraception (Table 1.11). Women who need effective contraception, who like to separate contraception from coitus, and who have a predictable schedule and can consistently take daily medication do well with OCPs. OCPs have a variety of noncontraceptive benefits (Table 1.11).

T ABLE 1.11. Noncontraceptive benefits of OCPs

Decrease risk of pelvic inflammatory disease by 50%
Improvement of fibrocystic disease of breasts
Decrease incidence and improvement in functional cysts of ovary
Increase in bone mass density in patients with primary and secondary amenorrhea
Decrease in breast cancer in long-term OCP users
Decrease in epithelial ovarian cancer incidence
Decrease in risk for endometrial cancer

Abbreviation: OCP, oral contraceptive pills.

T ABLE 1.12. Managing problems with women using OCPs

Problem	Comments	Questions	Management
CNS—headaches	Most are unrelated to OCPs	Evaluation of headache important	Occasionally may be caused by fluid retention, and use of OCP with lower estrogen may help. If headaches continue, D/C OCP
Depression	Most episodes are unrelated to OCP	Evaluate and treat depression	Switching to lower progestational OCP may decrease fatigue and tiredness
Hot flushes	Uncommon because estrogen dose is very high even in low-dose pills	Do they occur in week-off active hormones?	Woman may be going through menopause and needs to switch to HRT
		Do they occur during other 3 weeks?	Try OCP with higher-level estrogen
Acne	Usually caused by androgen activity	Think about polycystic ovary disease	Try OCP with less androgenic activity
Telangiectasias	Usually caused by increased estrogen levels	Think about liver diseases	Switch to OCP with lower estrogenic activity
Chloasma	May be caused by increased melanocyte stimulating hormone, caused by high estrogen levels		Switch to OCP with lower estrogenic activity; even so, this may be permanent
Hair loss	Usually not associated with OCP use, unless male pattern baldness		Try OCP with less androgenic activity. Rule out hypothyroid disease
Hirsuitism	Not uncommon	Think about polycystic ovary disease	Try OCP with less androgenic activity
Weight gain	OCPs on average do not increase weight	OCPs with high progestational and androgenic activity more likely to increase weight	Try OCP with less androgenic or progestational activity
Bloating	May be caused by progestins		Switch to OCP with lower estrogenic or progestational activity
Nausea/vomiting	Often decreases in time after first months		Take pills with food or at bedtime; if persists, try OCPs with lower estrogenic activity
Vaginal BTB	Most common in first few cycles and on low-dose OCPs; more common in smokers	Were pills missed?	Rule out pregnancy! Urge regular use
		First three cycles?	Try to continue—this will usually improve

continued

T ABLE 1.12. *continued* Managing problems with women using OCPs

Problem		Questions	Management
		Any chance pregnant?	Rule out pregnancy
		Continuing BTB in first half of cycle?	Switch to OCP with higher endometrial or progestational activity (see Table 1.13)
		BTB in second half of cycle?	Switch to OCP with higher progestational activity (Table 1.13)
Menorrhagia	Usually caused by insufficient progestin or excessive estrogen	Regular and just at time of menses?	Yes—switch to OCP with higher progestational and androgenic or lower endometrial activity
Oligomenorrhea	Usually caused by low-dose estrogen		Switch to higher endometrial activity OCP
Amenorrhea	Usually caused by low-dose estrogen		Rule out pregnancy; switch to higher endometrial activity OCP

Abbreviations: BTB, break-through-bleeding; CNS, central nervous system; HRT, hormone replacement therapy; OCPs, oral contraceptive pills.

- **Cost/availability.** The cost of OCPs is approximately $25 per month, plus an office visit at least annually.
- **Contraindications.** There are specific absolute and relative contraindications to estrogen-containing OCPs (Tables 1.3 and 1.4). Some medications should be avoided or used with caution in women who use OCPs.
- **Problems and side effects.** OCPs have a variety of side effects, some of which are common and innocent and some of which herald difficulties (Table 1.12). The most up-to-date, complete, and easiest-to-use source for this information is Dickey's *Managing Contraceptive Pill Patients* (EMIS Publishers, 1998, 9th ed.). Many common side effects can be managed by continuing the pills or switching to another pill, although there is no clinical evidence that changing the type or brand of pill effectively changes the side effect.

  Women who have BTB with one pill should change to one with a higher estrogenic potential (Table 1.13). If the BTB is late in the cycle, just before the monthly bleeding, a pill with a higher progestin activity may be tried. If breast tenderness, nausea, or acne is a problem, a pill with a second- or third-generation progestin or one with a lower progestin activity should be used (Table 1.13). Pills with high androgenic activity, such as Ovral and Lo/Ovral, worsen acne and facial hair. Certain side effects and symptoms make immediate cessation of OCPs necessary (Table 1.14).
- **STD protection.** No protection against any form of STD.

Progestin-Only Oral Contraceptives

Three progestin-only OCPs are available: Micronor, Nor QD (0.35 µg of norethindrone), and Ovrette (norgestrel). They must be taken at the same hour every day because of the low dose. The change in cervical mucus these pills induce may last only 22 hours.

- **Efficacy.** The efficacy of progestin-only OCPs is less than that of combination OCPs. The failure rate is 1% to 9% with usual use. The failure rate may be as much as 10 times higher in younger women (Fig. 1.4).

T ABLE 1.13. OCPs Ranked by endometrial and progestational activity*

High Endometrial Activity
Ovral
Lo-Ovral
Ovcon 50
Ortho-Novum 1/50; Norinyl 1/50
Ovcon 35

Medium Endometrial Activity
Ortho-cept; Ortho-Cyclen
Levlen
Ovcon 35
Ortho-Novum 1/35; Norinyl 1/35

Low Endometrial Activity
Tri-Norinyl
Estrostep
Ovrette
Micronor
Brevicon
Loestrin 1.5/30
Alesse
Demulen

High Progestational Activity
Ovral
Norlestrin 1/50
Demulen 50
Ortho-Cept
Loestrin 1.5/30
Demulen
Estrostep

Middle Progestational Activity
Ortho-Novum or Norinyl 1/50 or 1/35
Ovcon 50
Lo-Ovral
Levlen/Nordette
Ortho-Novum 7/7/7
Jenest
Trinorinyl

Low Progestational Activity
Ortho-Cyclen
Brevicon
Ortho Tri-Cyclen
Tri-Levlen/Triphasil
Ovcon 35
Alesse

*Pills with higher endometrial activity cause less breakthrough bleeding and more estrogen side effects.

T ABLE 1.14. Danger signs for women on OCPs

Symptom	Possible Emergent Condition Requiring Investigation
Loss or change in vision	Retinal artery thrombosis
Dysarthria, numbness	CVA
Change of consciousness	CVA
New-onset seizures	CVA
Leg swelling, redness, heat	DVT
Pulmonary (shortness of breath, hemoptysis)	PE
Breast mass	Cancer
Continuing heavy vaginal bleeding	Pregnancy, endometrial cancer
Amenorrhea	Pregnancy
RUQ abdominal pain, mass, or tenderness	Cholelithiasis, hepatitis, hepatoma

Abbreviations: CVA, cerebrovascular accident; DVT, deep venous thrombosis; PE, pulmonary embolism; RUQ, right upper quadrant.

- **Indications.** Progestin-only OCPs are a good choice for women who are breast-feeding; these pills may have some positive impact on breast milk production. They are a good choice, if pills are used at all, in women who smoke and are over 35 years of age. Women who are more than 45, who have had problems with estrogen side effects, or who have had DVT or hyperlipidemia may do well on these pills. There has been no measurable impact on the coagulation; however, the package insert still suggests that these be avoided in women with DVT or thrombotic events.
- **Cost/availability.** OCPs cost approximately $25 per month, plus an annual office visit.
- **Contraindications.** Women taking these pills often have BTB. Up to 40% of women taking progestin-only OCPs have irregular cycles. They may induce ovarian cysts; thus women who have problems with recurrent cysts may want to use a combination pill. These should be avoided in women receiving chronic rifampin (Rifadin) or anticonvulsants. Because of the low dose, any diminution by liver changes would likely inactivate the pill.

Injectable Progestin

DMP or Depo-Provera was widely studied for 30 years throughout the world before the U.S. Food and Drug Administration approved its use. It is an injectable form of progestin that lasts 14 weeks and is injected every 3 months at a dose of 150 mg IM. Unlike progestin implants (Norplant; see later), which release moderate long-term progesterone doses, Depo-Provera has high intermittent doses. It is thought to work by thickening cervical mucus and altering endometrium, and blocking the luteinizing hormone surge and ovulation. It must be injected within the first 5 days of the menstrual cycle.

- **Efficacy.** It has a very high efficacy rate of 99.7%, with fewer than three pregnancies per 1,000 women/years.
- **Indications.** It is a good choice for women with erratic lives or those who cannot remember to take pills (Table 1.15).
- **Cost/availability.** The shots cost $35 to $45 each, and most health providers require one yearly visit and quarterly pregnancy tests that add to the expense.
- **Contraindications.** Absolute contraindications include pregnancy and, because of this, unexplained vaginal bleeding (Table 1.16). Liver disease, breast cancer, and cardiovascular disease are relative contraindications. Because it takes longer to return to fertility after discontinuation of Depo-Provera than with OCPs, this may not be a good choice in women who want a quick return to fertility. Some reports have linked Depo-Provera with depression. However, none of these studies has investigated preuse psychiatric or psychologic state.
- **STD prevention.** None.

T ABLE 1.15. Women for whom Depo-Provera is a good choice

Breastfeeding women
Teenagers
Women whose lives are erratic—odd schedules, much travel
Women who forget to take daily pills
Women on anticonvulsants or antipsychotic medications
Women for whom estrogen is contraindicated—women with congenital heart disease, with thrombotic events, over 35 and a smoker, with hyperlipidemia

T ABLE 1.16. Contraindications to Depo-Provera and Norplant

	Depo-Provera	Norplant
Absolute		
Liver disease or cancer	No	Yes
Breast cancer	Yes	Yes
Pregnancy	Yes	Yes
Unexplained vaginal bleeding	Yes	Yes
Thrombotic disease	??	Yes
Relative		
Smoker older than 35	No	Possibly
Diabetes	No	No
Hyperlipidemia	Possibly	Possibly
Gallstones	No	No
Acne	Yes	Possibly
Migraine headaches	No	No
Depression	Yes?	Yes?
Medications using liver metabolism	No	Yes

Implantable Progestins

Norplant (six rod-shaped capsules of levonorgestrel) provides low-dose, long-acting hormonal contraception. Once placed, it gives very effective contraception for 5 years. It must be replaced after 5 years. Norplant works by inhibiting the luteinizing hormone (LH) surge and ovulation, making cervical mucus inimical, and causing endometrial atrophy. The method of insertion is easy to learn and all equipment is available in the insertion set. However, there have been difficulties with removal, causing this method to fall somewhat out of general favor. After removal of a Norplant, resumption of ovulatory cycles occurs rapidly, often within 1 month. Implanon, a single-rod, implantable progestin is just being made available.

- **Efficacy.** Norplant has a very high efficacy rate and almost no human failure. Fewer than two pregnancies per 1,000 women/years occur in women using Norplant. Most failures are from very early pregnancies present at the time of insertion; pregnancy tests and/or insertion only after a normal menstrual period can prevent these. Heavier women may experience slightly higher failure rates in the fourth and fifth years (Fig. 1.4).
- **Indications.** Norplant may be a good choice for women who cannot use estrogen-containing hormonal methods. The low daily dose avoids many troublesome side effects of OCPs. It is a good choice for women who do not or cannot take daily medication or do not want to use barrier methods. This is a good choice for women who may not be ready for sterilization but have completed their childbearing, barring accidents and remarriage. This is an excellent choice for women who for physical, medical, or occupational reasons should not get pregnant at all.
- **Cost/availability.** Norplant sets cost $250 to $300, with insertion costing between $150 and $300. Removal costs $150 to $350, but there are no other costs for 5 years. The physician and patient should be aware that insurance plans that pay for insertion may not be in effect to pay for removal when the time comes or may not pay for removal before 5 years, unless the physician certifies that it is medically

T ABLE 1.17. Medications that can be used to remedy breakthrough bleeding or menorrhagia while on Norplant or Depo-Provera

Nonsteroidal anti-inflammatory medications
  Naprosyn 375 mg PO bid or tid for 7 to 10 days
  Ibuprofen 800 mg PO bid or tid for 7 to 10 days
Estrogen
  Conjugated estrogens (Ortho-Est, Ogen) 1.25 mg PO qd for 7 days
  Estradiol 2 mg PO qd for 7 days
Combined oral contraceptives
Ortho-Novum or Norinyl, 1/35 or 1/50; Ortho-Cyclen or Tri-Cyclen, or Tri-Norinyl, or others for 3 weeks (the 3 weeks of active pills)

necessary. However, the manufacturer has a program for free insertion and removal for indigent women.
- **Contraindications.** Some women should not consider Norplant (Table 1.16). Two major problems with Norplant that have severely inhibited its use are irregular bleeding and difficulty in removal. Irregular bleeding occurs in as many as 8 out of 10 users. This is worse in the first year of use. BTB and menorrhagia occur very often and may be prolonged. Amenorrhea can occur. The woman and physician can minimize this irregular bleeding by use of nonsteroidal anti-inflammatory drugs (NSAIDs), estrogen, or combination OCPs for short periods. Some women do not find the amenorrhea acceptable (Table 1.17).

  Difficulty with removal has made physicians and patients less likely to use Norplant. Partially dependent on the insertion techniques and weight gain during the time since insertion, removal can be difficult and time-consuming. However, most removals are not painful, and 80% can be completed on the first try within 20 to 30 minutes, with only local anesthesia. However, the physician should see the video (provided by Wyeth) and practice on models beforehand. Other reported side effects include weight change, mastalgia, increased acne, and depression.
- **STD protection.** None.

Intrauterine devices (IUDs)

A variety of IUDs were on the market in the 1960s and 1970s, only one of which was the Dalkon Shield. This IUD used a multifiber string, and many pelvic infections and sterility occurred. A recall was suggested and most IUDs were taken off the U.S. market in the 1980s. Today the only IUDs available in the United States are Progestasert, a T-shaped IUD that releases progesterone and must be replaced yearly, and Paraguard, which can be used for 5 to 10 years. The progesterone IUD works by creating a spermicidal atmosphere within the uterine cavity, inhibiting implantation and creating inimical cervical mucus. Once the IUD is removed, the woman can immediately become pregnant; there is no prolonged wait for return to fertility.
- **Efficacy.** IUDs have a pregnancy rate of approximately 1% to 2%, with a 2% to 3% expulsion rate, and a 10% removal rate yearly.
- **Indications.** IUDs are indicated for women who want to space their pregnancies, avoid taking pills or having to remember pills, and avoid hormonal effects but are not yet ready for sterilization.
- **Cost/availability.** The IUD set costs between $150 and $200. Insertion costs approximately $50 to $125. Removal usually costs no more than an office visit.

24WOMEN'S HEALTH

- **Contraindications.** Nulliparous women, women who have had pelvic inflammatory disease (PID) or infections, and women with multiple partners or abnormally shaped uteruses should not use an IUD.
- **Side effects.** Pregnancy with IUDs is rare, but IUDs do not prevent tubal implantation, although they do not increase the risk of tubal pregnancy. If an IUD user becomes pregnant, the chance that the pregnancy is ectopic is increased. An ultrasound to determine placement of the pregnancy is mandatory.

  Spontaneous Abortion If a woman has an intrauterine pregnancy with an IUD in place, the chance of spontaneous abortion is 60%. If the IUD is removed immediately, the chance of spontaneous abortion drops to 30%. If a woman becomes pregnant, the IUD should be removed.

  Menorrhagia Women who use IUDs often mention increased menstrual bleeding and dysmenorrhea. The newer IUDs are more likely to decrease the amount of menstrual bleeding and have far less dysmenorrhea, although this may be worse in the first few months.

  Pelvic Infection Risk of pelvic infection is higher in the first 20 days after insertion, but rare afterward.

- **STD protection.** None.

Sterilization

Female Sterilization

Female sterilization is the most common form of sterilization worldwide and in the United States. It can be accomplished by a hysterectomy. However, it is primarily achieved by one of a variety of methods of tubal ligation (TL). TL can be done immediately postpartum (as 50% of TLs are) or any other time. Although tuboplasties with subsequent successful pregnancies are possible, the woman and the physician should consider TL in any form permanent. Thus it should be only used when the woman has finished childbearing.

- **Efficacy.** TL has almost no human error. Postpartum failure rates are 1 in 250 pregnancies and are caused by recanalization. TLs done at other times have a failure rate of 1 in 400 procedures, mostly caused by very early (<2-week-old) gestations at the time of the procedure (Fig. 1.4).
- **Indications.** Permanent contraception is the indication for sterilization.
- **Cost/availability.** Cost varies from approximately $1,200 to $2,500, including the physician's and anesthesiologist's fee and operating room time. However, it is a one-time cost and is usually covered by insurance.
- **Contraindications.** Contraindications include any chance that the woman or couple may wish to have children in the future. Women may have menstrual changes after the TL.
- **STD protection.** None.

Male Sterilization

Approximately 7% to 12% of couples use male sterilization, primarily vasectomy.
- **Efficacy.** Failure rate is less than one in 400 procedures (Fig. 1.4).
- **Indications.** The couple should desire permanent sterility.
- **Cost/availability.** Male sterilization can be done in outpatient surgery and costs between $250 and $1,200. It is often covered by insurance.
- **Contraindications.** Any desire for future children. Vasectomy does not increase the likelihood of coronary artery disease or myocardial infarctions.
- **STD protection.** None.

SPECIAL POPULATIONS

Adolescents

Sixty percent of teenagers do not use contraceptives at their first sexual experience, and there may be an average period of 18 months between the first sexual encounter and use of contraception. A teenage girl 15 years of age or younger in the United States is four times more likely to become pregnant than in the United Kingdom, Canada, France, the Netherlands, and Sweden, although rates of teenage sexual activity are similar. In the United States, girls younger than 15 years of age are more likely to use condoms than are older girls, and boys are more likely to use condoms and withdrawal, if any contraception is used. Encouragingly, the rate of condom use among teenagers is increasing, almost doubling from 1982 to 1988.

Appropriate Methods

Appropriate methods include the following (Table 1.18):
- Abstinence may be the most appropriate method of contraception.
- Condoms are a very good choice, particularly for couples who are not in long-term relationships and are not monogamous. They are needed for prevention of STDs in this population especially.
- Spermicides, especially when used with condoms, can be effective and can be acceptable to adolescents.
- Most hormonal methods of contraception are appropriate and can be used very effectively and agreeably by teenagers. OCPs, DMP, Norplant, and EC can be used. Although they can be used, OCPs with progestins that have a high androgenic component—specifically norgestrel (Ovral, Lo/Ovral) and progestin-only OCPs—may be less appealing to teenagers because they may cause or worsen acne and hair changes. DMP may be preferred because of ease of administration and the amenorrhea that occurs after a few doses. EC may be appropriate and acceptable for the lifestyles of teenagers. Teenagers must be educated about its existence and how to obtain a health provider appointment or the pills. EC use provides an opportunity to counsel and offer suggestions for a long-term contraceptive method.

Inappropriate Methods

- Rhythm and NFP are not good methods for adolescents because girls of this age often have irregular periods.
- CI is not a good method for adolescents because teenagers' speed of ejaculation and lack of control decrease its efficacy.

T ABLE 1.18. Choice of contraception in adolescents

Good Methods	Acceptable Choices	Poor Choices
Abstinence	Diaphragms	Rhythm or NFP
EC	Norgestrel-containing OCPs	IUD
Condoms, male or female		Coitus interruptus
Spermicides		Sterilization
OCPs		
Norplant		
Depo-Provera		

Abbreviations: EC, emergency contraception; IUD, intrauterine device; OCPs, oral contraceptive pills; NFP, natural family planning.

- Many adolescents lack the experience and comfort to use diaphragms effectively.
- IUDs are contraindicated in nulliparous women because they may produce infections that can produce sterility or infertility.
- Sterilization is not a good option for teenagers.

Breastfeeding Women

Appropriate Methods

Appropriate methods include the following (Table 1.19):
- Any lack-of-contact or barrier method may be used during breastfeeding.
- Progestin-containing hormonal methods—progestin-only OCPs, Norplant, or DMP—can be used. Norplant and progestin-only OCPs should not be used before 6 weeks postpartum. Although there are anecdotal reports of DMP affecting breast milk production, it can be given immediately postpartum.
- IUDs can be used.
- Sterilization can be used.

Inappropriate Methods

Because menstrual periods may be absent or irregular, rhythm or NFP may not be a good choice for the breastfeeding mother.
- Some hormonal methods of contraception may impede successful breastfeeding or be excreted in the breast milk. Specifically, estrogen-containing OCPs should be avoided.

Older Women

Appropriate Methods

Except for smokers, almost any method is appropriate for older women and acceptable, depending on the woman and couple.
- CI may be very effective in older couples.
- Barrier methods are acceptable.
- Hormonal methods (except in smokers, women with a history of thromboembolic disease, or other contraindications) are permissible. Older women may use progestin-only OCPs to avoid the effects or problems with estrogen.
- IUDs, especially long-term ones, may be a good choice.
- Sterilization may be an acceptable method of contraception for women who have completed childbearing.

T ABLE 1.19. Contraceptive choices for breastfeeding women

Good Choices	Acceptable Choices	Poor Choices
Abstinence	CI	NFP or rhythm
Condom, spermicide	Sterilization	EC
Diaphragms		Estrogen-containing OCPs
IUD		
Progestin-only OCPs		
DMP		
Norplant*		
Sterilization		

Abbreviations: CI, coitus interruptus; DMP, depomedroxyprogesterone; EC, emergency contraception; IUD, intrauterine device; OCPs, oral contraceptive pills; NFP, natural family planning.
*Wait 6 weeks postpartum.

Inappropriate Methods

- Lack-of-contact methods, especially NFP, may work well for long-term monogamous couples. However, menstrual periods may become irregular nearing menopause, which makes this method more difficult.
- Women who are older than age 35 and smoke may not use estrogen-containing OCPs.

Disabled Women

Depending on the disability, the couple may have to modify their choice of contraception (Table 1.20).

- Women who have mechanical difficulties (e.g., amputations, muscular problems, multiple sclerosis, cerebral palsy, strokes, or myasthenia gravis) may want to use hormonal contraception or sterilization. Use of condoms, especially female condoms, or a diaphragm may be difficult. It may also be difficult for women with these disabilities to check for IUD strings.

T ABLE 1.20. Contraception methods for women with disabilities

Disability	Good	Acceptable	Poor
		Quality	
Amputation	NFP or rhythm, progestin-only OCPs, Norplant, sterilization	OCPs (unless at high risk of DVTs), EC, condoms, spermicides	Female condom, diaphragm, IUD
Blindness or visual impairment	OCPs, DMP, Norplant, IUD, EC, sterilization	Male condom	Female condom, spermicides, rhythm
CVA or cerebral palsy	Progestin-only OCPs, EC, Norplant, DMP, NFP, or rhythm	Male condom	Female condom, spermicides, diaphragm, IUD, estrogen-containing OCPs
Epilepsy	OCPs,* DMP, Norplant, EC, diaphragm, sterilization	Condom, spermicides, NFP or rhythm*	
Muscular diseases, multiple sclerosis, or arthritis	NFP or rhythm, OCPs, DMP, Norplant, EC, sterilization	Male condom	Female condom, spermicides, IUD, diaphragm
Spinal cord injury or wheelchair-bound	NFP or rhythm, DMP, Norplant, EC, sterilization	Male condom	Female condom, spermicides, IUD, diaphgram, estrogen-containing OCPs (except third generation: may increase risk of DVTs)

Abbreviations: CVA, cerebrovascular accident; DMP, depomedroxyprogesterone; DVT, deep venous thrombosis; EC, emergency contraception; IUD, intrauterine device; NFP, natural family planning; OCPs, oral contraceptive pills.

*Watch antiepileptic drug levels.

- Women who are confined to wheelchairs may want to avoid estrogen-containing hormonal preparations or use a third-generation OCP to decrease the risk of DVTs.
- Women with epilepsy can take hormonal medication but may need to watch the levels of antiseizure medications. Anticonvulsant medications can interfere with regularity of menstrual periods, making rhythm and NFP less effective.
- Women who have a visual disability may have trouble using condoms, spermicides, and rhythm.

SUGGESTED READING

Cancer and Steroid Hormone Study of the Centers for Disease Control and the National Institute of Child Health and Human Development. Oral contraceptive use and the risk of breast cancer. *N Engl J Med* 1986;315:405.

Colditz GA. Oral contraceptive use and mortality during 12 years of follow-up. The Nurses' Health Study. *Ann Intern Med* 1994;120:821.

Goldfarb L, Gerrard M, Gibbons FX, Plante T. Attitudes toward sex, arousal, and the retention of contraceptive information. *J Pers Soc Psychol* 1988;55:634.

Knopp RH, La Rosa JC, Burkman R. Contraception and dyslipidemia. *Am J Obstet Gynecol* 1993;168:1994.

Speroff L, Darney W. *A clinical guide to contraception.* Baltimore: Williams & Wilkins, 1996.

Speroff L, DeCherney A. Evaluation of a new generation of oral contraceptives. *Obstet Gynecol* 1993;81:1034.

Ursin G, Ross RK, Sullivan HJ. Use of oral contraceptives and risk of breast cancer in young women. *Breast Cancer Res Treat* 1998;50:175.

WHO Collaborative Study of Cardiovascular Disease and Steroid Hormone Contraception. Venous thromboembolic disease and combined oral contraceptives. *Lancet* 1995;348:1575.

CHAPTER 2

Gynecologic Cancers

Jo Ann Rosenfeld and Rick Kellerman

Cancers in the female reproductive tract most commonly include cervical, endometrial, and ovarian cancers. The first is preventable, and the first two are usually curable. Unfortunately, ovarian cancer is often discovered only after it has already metastasized and it is too late for cure. Prevention, detection, and treatment of these cancers concern women of all ages.

CERVICAL CANCER

Chief Complaints
- A 24-year-old woman has human papillomavirus (HPV) changes on her yearly Pap smear.
- A 36-year-old woman has cervical intraepithelial neoplasia (CIN II) on her Pap smear, and this is confirmed on colposcopy.
- A 54-year-old postmenopausal woman who has not had a Pap smear in 24 years comes in complaining of the sudden onset of vaginal bleeding.

Clinical Manifestations
- Usually none
- Sometimes vaginal bleeding, cramping
- Menometrorrhagia
- Vaginal discharge
- Pain, weight loss, constipation, diarrhea, and/or urinary tract infections (UTIs) (late in the disease)

Epidemiology
- Six percent of all cancers in women are gynecologic.
- An estimated 14,500 new cases of cervical cancer are diagnosed yearly in the United States.
- Rates have decreased steadily over the past decades, from 14.2 per 100,000 in 1973 to 8.2 per 100,000 in 1993.
- Cancer *in situ* (CIS) is more common than invasive cancer, particularly in women under 50 years of age. Approximately 50,000 new cases of cervical CIS are diagnosed yearly.
- Approximately 4,800 deaths due to cervical cancer occurred in 1997. In 1993 the death rate was almost half that in 1973.
- Cervical cancer rates in African Americans declined more rapidly than those in whites from 1973 to 1993 (Fig. 2.1). However, the mortality rate in African-American women in 1993 was still more than twice that in white women.

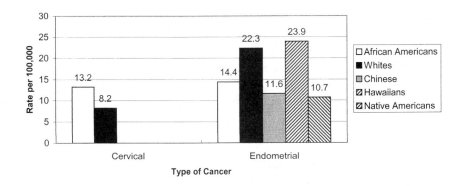

FIGURE 2.1. Incidence rate for cancers by ethnicity.

Risk Factors

Risk factors are outlined in Table 2.1.

Risky sexual behavior. The risk correlates with the number of sexual partners and the number of partners each partner has had. Early (before 18 years of age) first intercourse is also associated with a higher rate of cervical cancer.

The **increased incidence of HPV** is one of the most important reasons for the increase in precancerous lesions of the cervix. HPV is found in most (39%) cervical carcinomas and precursor lesions worldwide. Transmission is sexual. More than 40 subtypes are known. Types 16, 18, 31, 33, 35, 41, 45, 52, 56, and 58 are associated with cervical cancer and genital neoplasias, and they account for more than 80% of all invasive cervical cancers. HPV infection occurs in the cervical, vaginal, and perineal tissues. If one lesion is visible, other lesions are present. HPV can be transmitted even when condoms are used during sexual intercourse. Infection occurs most often in women 22 to 25 years of age. The prevalence of infection decreases with increasing age.

Presence of either **herpes simplex virus** (HSV) infection of genitalia (type 2) or **other sexually transmitted diseases** is also a risk factor.

Cigarette smoking and passive smoking. Women who smoke are three times more likely to develop cervical cancer precursors. The national history of premalig-

T ABLE 2.1.   Risk factors for cervical cancer

Never or seldom having a Pap test
Sexual behavior
    Increased number of sexual partners
    Early first intercourse
STD history
    HSV
    HPV
Cigarette smoking and passive smoking

HPV, human papillomavirus; HSV, herpes simplex virus; STD, sexually transmitted disease.

nant disease is influenced by smoking, relating to interference with immune system response.

Never having a Pap smear. This is the greatest risk factor for cervical cancer. A woman who has never had a Pap smear is 50 to 60 times more likely to have cervical cancer than a woman who has had one in the past 3 years. Half of cervical cancers in the United States occur in women who have never been screened.

Long-term use of oral contraceptive pills (OCPs) is also a risk factor.

Risk Reduction

The following are associated with reduced risk of cervical cancer:
- Use of barrier contraceptives and spermicides
- Condom use
- Avoidance of high-risk sexual activity
- Smoking cessation
- High dietary levels of vitamin C

Pathology

Cervical cancer arises from single-cell precursors in the transformation zone of the cervix.

Diagnosis

Pap Smear

A Pap smear should be performed in women more than 18 years of age or in those who are or have been sexually active. Use of the Pap smear for screening has reduced cervical cancer mortality by more than 70% (Fig. 2.2). Many women are missed. All populations should be screened. The primary reason for failure of eradication of invasive carcinoma of the cervix is not misdiagnosis, but a lack of screening. After 65 years of age, routine screening may be discontinued if findings are normal on two consecutive Pap smears. High-risk women should have annual screenings. Women who are at an increased risk include the following:
- Women with a previously abnormal Pap
- Women with condylomatous warts
- Women who are immunocompromised

After three or more normal results, the American Cancer Society and the American Academy of Family Physicians suggest that the Pap smear may be done less than yearly as decided by the physician. Other organizations have differing suggestions. Medicare pays for one Pap smear every 3 years.

A Pap smear has a high false-negative rate of 20% to 40%. The false-positive rate ranges from 0 to 8%. An adequate Pap smear has cells from the transformation zone and the endocervix. Use of an Ayres speculum with an endocervical nylon cytobrush usually produces an adequate specimen. The slide should be fixed immediately so that it does not dry out.

The Pap smear is reported using the 1991 Bethesda system, which lists three qualities (Figure 2.2):
I. Slide adequacy
    A. Satisfactory for evaluation.
    B. Satisfactory for evaluation but limited by the following:
        1. Lack of endocervical cells (ECC). If limited by lack of ECC, the Pap does not have to be repeated within 1 year. Lack of ECC can be caused by pregnancy, nulliparity, or atrophic mucosa, or it can follow an excisional treatment.
        2. Excessive mucus.

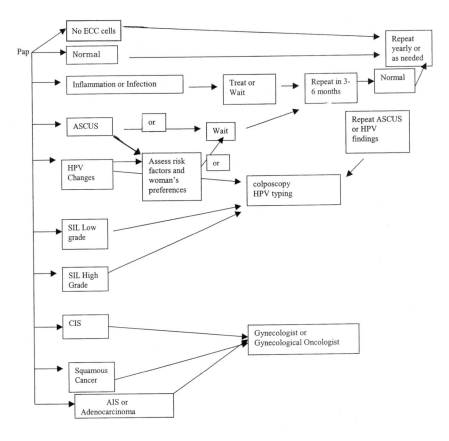

FIGURE 2.2. Evaluation of Pap smear results. ECC, endocervical cells; ASCUS, atypical squamous cells of undetermined significance; HPV, human papillomavirus; SIL, squamous intraepithelial lesion; CIS, cancer *in situ*; AIS, adenocarcinoma *in situ*.

       3. Inflammation, blood, or debris. The evaluation of a Pap smear with this report would be followed by culture, treatment, and a repeat in 8 to 12 weeks.

       4. Drying artifact—repeat.

       5. Lack of patient information—repeat.

    C. Unsatisfactory for evaluation.

II. Cellular description

    A. Normal.

    B. Benign cellular changes, including metaplasia (squamous metaplasia is the normal reparative and reactive process in which columnar epithelium, when exposed to liquids or air, becomes squamous) or atrophy. Atrophy is normal in postmenopausal women. These are normal findings and require no treatment.

    C. Epithelial cell abnormalities. These are either squamous or glandular. Squamous abnormalities have four categories:

1. Atypical squamous cells of undetermined significance (ASCUS). These cells are not inflammatory or koilocytotic atypia. These women can be watched because 5% to 30% (depending on population) of cases may be normal. On review, slightly less than 5% of slides are actually ASCUS and up to 75% of ASCUS are associated with normal histology. All women with ASCUS slides need a repeat Pap smear in 3 to 6 months. If it is still ASCUS, colposcopy is indicated.
2. Low-grade squamous intraepithelial lesion (LGSIL). This category includes cells with effects of HPV, including koilocytosis and mild dysplasia. All women with LGSIL should have colposcopy. Twenty-two percent to 78% of women with LGSIL have Pap tests that return to normal or regress in as little as 18 months. Fewer than 2% progress to cancer, and fewer than 16% worsen to high-grade squamous intraepithelial lesion (HGSIL). Usually three out of four cases will not progress, and 40% remain as LGSIL. Of those that progress, only 10% progress to CIS.
3. HGSIL. All women with Pap smear with HGSIL should have a colposcopy, and treatment depends on colposcopy findings.
4. CIS or squamous cancer. Women with CIS or squamous cancer should generally be referred immediately to a gynecologist or gynecologic oncologist.
   D. Glandular abnormalities. Women with atypical glandular cells (AGUS) need an ultrasound, colposcopy, and possibly cone excision.
III. Hormonal effect (or evaluation)
   A. Hormonal pattern compatible with age and history.

Evaluation

Colposcopy involves abnormal screening tests (Fig. 2.3). This procedure has been used since 1925, mostly in Europe, and gives a more accurate visual inspection of the cervix. Colposcopy is used to evaluate abnormalities found on the screening Pap test. The purpose is to find the most severely abnormal area on the cervix and biopsy that area. If the total transformation zone is seen and that area's pathology is the same as that on the Pap, and the pathologic area is totally on the exocervix, then local treatment is possible and cone excision is avoided. When used properly, 90% of conizations can be avoided. Thus the squamocolumnar junction and transformation zone must be visualized on the exocervix. The lesion must be identified on the exocervix. No higher-grade or severer lesion than that found on Pap can be identified. An endocervical curettage can always be performed to evaluate for endocervical lesions. If the curettage is positive, it indicates an endocervical lesion requiring cone excision.

Indications for Treatment

Treatment is determined based on colposcopy findings correlating with Pap test screening.
• **No correlation.** Referral for cone excision or conization.
• **Endocervical curettage positive.** Referral for cone excision.
• **Cervicitis, HPV findings, curettage negative.** Repeat Pap or colposcopy in 3 months, then every 3 months for 9 months.
• **LGSIL.** Watch patient for 3 months, triaged by risk and HPV type, or treat with cyrosurgery or loop excision electrosurgery procedure (LEEP). If the woman's risk is high or the likelihood of return visit is low, treatment may be indicated. Three-quarters of cases will return to normal or remain LGSIL.
• **HGSIL.** Treatment with cryosurgery or LEEP, or referral for laser surgery or cone excision.

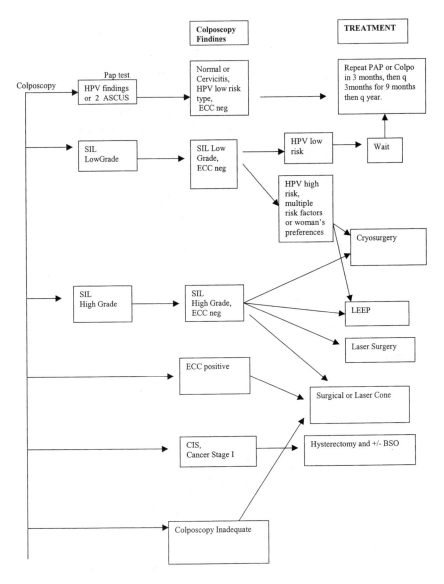

FIGURE 2.3. Evaluation of colposcopy findings. LEEP, loop excision electro-surgery procedure; BSO, bilateral salpingo-oopho-rectomy.

- **CIS.** Cone excision.
- **Cancer.** Referral for staging and appropriate therapy.

REFERRAL

Referral should be considered for patients with inadequate colposcopy findings, CIN III, CIS, or cancer.

Management

Cervical Dysplasia

Some studies suggest nutritional factors may influence resolution of cervical dysplasia. Supplements with folate, beta carotene, and vitamins A, C, and E may promote resolution of dysplasia. Note that use of condoms to prevent reinfection with HPV has not been shown to affect resolution of cervical dysplasia. Other possible management approaches include:

Smoking cessation (if the patient smokes).

Cryosurgery. This is inexpensive, easy to do, and quick; it has little morbidity, mortality, or effect on future reproduction. No anesthesia is necessary, except for local, if desired. A 3- to 4-mm "freezeball" must be obtained, usually by several repeated freezes. The only problem is that this is ablative, and no further cytology or histology can be done.

LEEP. It is indicated in exocervical disease, treatment of SIL in which squamocolumnar junction is visible, and when the transformation zone is entirely on the exocervix and the ECC is negative. Contraindications to LEEP are listed in Table 2.2. A 2- to 3-cm by 2-cm block, including most of the transformation zone, is excised by loop electrocautery. The benefits to LEEP are that it provides a histologic specimen for pathologic examination and margins can be determined. It can be done in the office in 15 to 30 minutes. It requires cervical anesthesia with lidocaine or paracervical block. It has been reported to have little affect on future childbearing. There is a 4% rate of excessive bleeding. LEEP leaves no devitalized tissue behind.

Cone excision. This can be done by laser, liquid carbon dioxide, or "cold" knife surgical conization. This can affect future childbearing and is usually done in a surgical suite by a gynecologist or gynecologic oncologist.

Both cone excision and LEEP produce samples of similar cone depth, but depth of thermal injury is increased in laser cone conization. The laser does more damage to cervical tissues and has greater mean operating time.

Laser surgery has complications. Immediate ones are bleeding and infection. Long-term complications include an increased risk of preterm birth following cervical laser procedures.

CIS. *In situ* cancer can be treated with cryotherapy, laser excision, LEEP, or surgical cone excision.

Invasive Cancers

Invasive cancers are treated by surgery or radiation.

TABLE 2.2. Contraindications to LEEP

Pregnancy
Suspected invasive disease of cervix
Acute cervicitis
Bleeding disorder
Inadequate colposcopy

Abbreviation: LEEP, loop excision electrosurgery procedure.

T ABLE 2.3. International Federation of Gynecologists and Obstetricians staging system for cervical cancer, 1994

Stage	Description
0	Carcinoma *in situ,* intraepithelial carcinoma
I	Carcinoma confined to cervix
IA	Identifiable only microscopically
IB	Gross lesions or lesion with stromal invasion > 7 mm
II	Carcinoma beyond the cervix but not extended to pelvic wall
III	Extension to pelvic wall, hydronephrosis
IV	Extension beyond the true pelvis

Survival is based on stage (Table 2.3). In patients with cervical cancer, the survival rate at 1 year is 87%; at 5 years it is 69% (Fig. 2.4).

If detected early, invasive cervical cancer has a 5-year survival rate of 91%. White women are more likely than African-American women to have their cervical cancer identified early. Fifty-five percent of white and 39% of African-American women's cancers are diagnosed at this stage.

Stage 0 disease or microinvasion of less than 3 mm is highly curable with either simple hysterectomy or cone biopsy with clear margins for women wanting fertility. Patients with stage I and IA disease have a 70% to 85% cure rate with either radical surgery or radiation. Higher stages of disease are treated with radiation. The 5-year survival rate is 40% to 60%.

The depth of stromal invasion is clearly linked to the risk of nodal involvement, cancer recurrence, and mortality. As depth of invasion increases, so does the risk of nodal disease. With invasion of up to 3 mm, risk of nodal disease was 1.9% and mortality was under 1%; beyond 3 mm, the risk of nodal involvement is 7.8%. Lesions that penetrate the basement membrane by up to 1 mm were associated with lymphatic vascular space invasion, and this increases fivefold when the basement membrane was penetrated 3 to 5 mm.

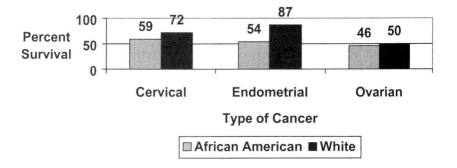

FIGURE 2.4. Relative 5-year cancer survival rate by race.

Follow-up

A repeat Pap test after treatment for cervical dysplasia should occur every 3 months for 1 year, and then yearly.

Follow-up after hysterectomy for CIS or stage I cancer should be yearly.

ENDOMETRIAL CANCER

Chief Complaint

- A 54-year-old postmenopausal woman with new-onset vaginal bleeding.
- A 68-year-old woman with new onset of recurrent urinary tract infection (UTI).

Clinical Manifestations

- Usually none
- Abnormal uterine bleeding, cramping (75% of cases occur in postmenopausal women who present with abnormal vaginal bleeding and thus are detected at an early stage)
- Cramping
- Late symptoms: pain, weight loss, constipation, and recurrent UTIs

Epidemiology

- An estimated 34,900 new cases diagnosed yearly. Rates have stayed steady at 21/100,000 women.
- Endometrial cancer is the fourth most common malignancy in women and the seventh most common cause of cancer death in women.
- Endometrial cancer caused an estimated 600 deaths in 1997. Mortality rates are 3/100,000.
- Endometrial cancer is more common in African-Americans and Hawaiians (Fig. 2.1).

Risk Factors

Table 2.4 lists risk factors for endometrial cancer.
- Most cancers occur in women who have had endogenous or exogenous unopposed estrogen.

T ABLE 2.4. Risk factors for endometrial cancer

Estrogen excess
    Hormone replacement with unopposed estrogen
    Early menarche
    Late menopause
    Never having children
    History of failure to ovulate
    Stein-Leventhal syndrome
    Obesity
Tamoxifen use
Associated medical conditions
    Diabetes
    Gallbladder disease
    Hypertension

- Endometrial cancer is associated with obesity (caused by peripheral conversion of androstenendione to estrone by extra glandular aromatization in adipose tissues), Stein-Leventhal syndrome, or estrogen-producing tumors such as granulosa cell tumors of the ovary.
- Estrogen replacement therapy (ERT) or unopposed estrogen administration is associated with a four- to eightfold increased risk of endometrial cancer, and these cases are predominantly early-stage, low-grade, minimally invasive lesions with favorable prognosis. This increased risk is negated by combining progesterone with estrogen.
- Tamoxifen use is a risk factor for endometrial cancer. Tamoxifen is an antiestrogen that is used in breast cancer patients. It has been linked to endometrial cancer. Use of tamoxifen gives a 6.4-fold increased risk of endometrial cancer.
- Other causes of increased exposure to estrogen during life include early menarche, late (after 52 years of age) menopause, never having children, and history of failure to ovulate.
- Other medical conditions have been linked to increased risk of endometrial cancer, including diabetes, gallbladder disease, hypertension, and obesity.
- Pregnancy and use of OCPs help reduce the risk of endometrial cancer.

Pathology

Endometrial columnar cells become cancerous.

Diagnosis

A proposed approach to diagnosis is shown in Fig. 2.5.
- Pap smears are not effective for detecting early endometrial cancer.
- In the postmenopausal woman with abnormal bleeding, ultrasound (with measurement of the endometrial stripe) and endometrial biopsy or dilation and curettage (D&C) provide sufficient information to evaluate for cancer.
- Ultrasound alone, if the endometrial stripe is less than 5 mm, may be sufficient to eliminate endometrial cancer. Most women with endometrial cancer had an endometrial stripe of more than 14 mm. The best studies show this in postmenopausal women.
- Endometrial biopsy, if positive, confirms endometrial cancer. A negative result does not eliminate endometrial cancer as a cause for postmenopausal bleeding and D&C or hysterectomy with biopsy should follow.
- A negative histologic report from a D&C does rule out cancer.

Referral

Referral may be indicated for a diagnostic D&C, endometrial biopsy (if not performed by a family physician), or definitive hysterectomy.

Management

- **Low-risk patients, stage IA.** Treatment includes surgery (including sampling of peritoneal fluid), total abdominal hysterectomy (TAH), and bilateral salpingo-oophorectomy (BSO). These patients do not benefit from postoperative radiation.
- **Patients at intermediate risk, IB or II.** After surgery, adjuvant pelvic radiation is of questionable benefit in this group and provides no improved survival.
- **Patients at high risk of recurrence.** Those patients with extrauterine disease benefit from adjuvant therapy. Postoperatively, whole-pelvis radiation is beneficial.
- **Patients with abdominal metastasis.** These patients may also need chemotherapy.

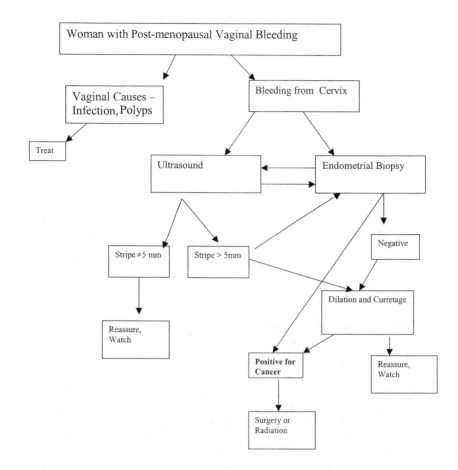

FIGURE 2.5. Evaluation of postmenopausal bleeding.

Follow-Up

- Postoperative surveillance guidelines: If the woman has no postoperative evidence of disease, then follow-up every 3 months for 2 years, then every 6 months for 3 years is indicated, including a complete examination of breasts, abdomen, and pelvis and Pap (although used, it seldom changes therapy). Chest x-rays do not improve survival rates. However, many experts suggest a chest x-ray annually for 3 years after surgery.
- Fourteen percent of patients develop recurrent disease.
- Can women with stage I endometrial cancer who have had TAH with BSO take ERT? A small prospective study showed that women who had had surgery many years earlier and who took ERT had no increase in recurrence rates of endometrial cancer.
- Ninety-three percent of endometrial cancer patients survive 1 year (Table 2.5). If cancer is discovered at the regional stage, the 5-year survival rate is 66%. White women's survival rates exceeded those of African-American women by 15% at every stage.

T ABLE 2.5.   Staging of endometrial cancer

I. Carcinoma confined to the corpus
   IA. Uterine cavity is 8 cm or less
   IB. Depth of uterine cavity >8 cm
II. Carcinoma in corpus and cervix
III. Carcinoma outside uterus but not outside pelvis
IV. Carcinoma outside true pelvis or has involved mucosa of bladder or rectum

OVARIAN CANCER

The problem with ovarian cancer is that most women present with advanced disease. There are no effective screening tools, and genetic screening is not indicated for most women. The chance to detect and cure ovarian cancer occurs only if ovarian masses are thoroughly evaluated.

Chief Complaints
• An 82-year-old woman with new-onset shortness of breath and increasing abdominal mass
• A 63-year-old woman with recurrent UTIs
• A 23-year-old woman with abdominal pain and weight loss

Clinical Manifestations
• Usually none until disease is advanced.
• Occasionally, an enlarged ovary is detected on physical examination, or by chance on a radiologic or ultrasound study.
• Symptoms of abdominal and pleural metastases such as pain, constipation, fistulas, UTIs, ascites, increasing abdominal circumference, and shortness of breath occur late in the course.

Epidemiology
• Ovarian cancer is the fifth leading cause of cancer death in women and has the highest mortality of the gynecologic cancers.
• Twenty-five percent of patients present in stage I, but two-thirds present with advanced disease (Fig. 2.6).
• Most common in women older than 60 years of age.

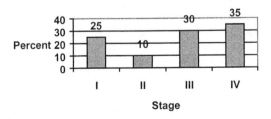

FIGURE 2.6.   Percentage stage presentation of ovarian cancers.

Risk Factors
- Women older than 60 years of age
- Low parity or nulliparous
- Family history of ovarian cancer

Risk Reduction
The following factors reduce the risk of ovarian cancer: childbearing, use of OCPs (as little as 6 months of use), breast-feeding, tubal sterilization.

Diagnosis
Differential diagnosis and evaluation of ovarian mass is dependent on the age and hormonal state of the patient (Fig. 2.7 and Table 2.6).

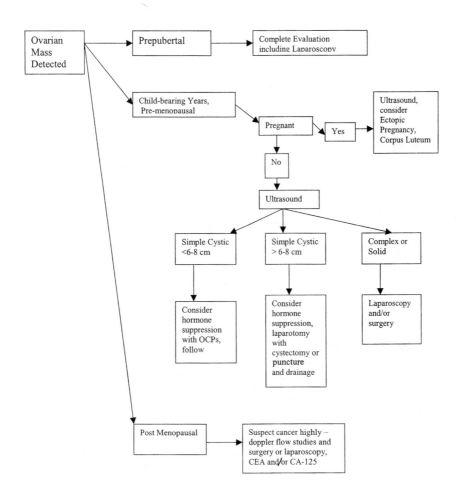

TABLE 2.6. Differential diagnosis of ovarian mass

Prepubertal
  Cancer
  Teratoma
Childbearing years
  Cancer
  Ectopic pregnancy
  Functional cyst
  Corpus luteum
  Tubo-ovarian abscess
  Serous or mucinous cystadenoma
    Teratoma
    Endometrioma
Postmenopausal
  Cancer
  Teratoma
  Abscess

Screening

Screening tests could include bimanual pelvic examination, Pap test, tumor marker, and ultrasound imaging.

- Pap test is of no value in screening for ovarian cancer.
- Bimanual pelvic examinations can occasionally detect ovarian cancer, but women in whom cancers are discovered by this method usually have advanced disease and poorer survival rates. Bimanual examinations have many false-positive results.
- Tumor markers include carcinoembryonic antigen (CEA), CA-125, and others. CA-125 is elevated in 82% of women with advanced disease and in many women with early disease. Sensitivity is 29% to 75% in stage I disease. Present evidence suggests that tumor markers do not become elevated early enough to detect disease at a curable stage. One-half of women who developed cancer of the ovary had elevated levels 1.5 to 3 years before diagnosis. Further research is needed to determine the reliability of tumor markers.
- Ultrasound evaluation (transvaginally or transabdominally) is 50% to 100% sensitive and 76% to 97% specific in detecting ovarian cancer. However, routine ultrasound evaluation to screen produces many false-positive results, leading to many unnecessary laparotomies. Even in women with previous breast or gynecologic cancer, screening of more than 5,500 women found only two ovarian cancers in more than 6,900 scans. The U.S. Preventive Services Task Force does not recommend routine screening by ultrasound. Screening for genetic predisposition is available but its use is limited.
- Fewer than 0.1% of women are affected by hereditary ovarian cancer, and these women have a lifetime risk of 40% of developing ovarian cancer.
- Women with a family member who has had ovarian cancer might consider asking that family members be screened for genetic syndromes (such as BRCA1 or 2). If the test result is positive, other family members can then be screened. Wide, unrestricted screening is not suggested at present.

Follow-Up

- Overall 5-year survival rate is 75% if cancer is confined to the ovaries, and 17% if diagnosed when metastasis has occurred.
- After TAH and BSO, further adjuvant therapy is dependent on the stage. Stage IA and IB grade I tumors do not require adjuvant therapy. Most women with stage IC and higher-grade tumors benefit from added chemotherapy, especially if they have clear cell carcinoma.

C HAPTER 3

Breast Disease

Jo Ann Rosenfeld

Breast cancer (BCa) is the most prevalent form of cancer in women and a major cause of cancer mortality. However, if it is detected early, it is curable. Screening can reduce mortality in some populations.

CHIEF COMPLAINTS

- A 35-year-old woman with multiple tender nodules in both breasts
- A 56-year-old woman with a small, hard nodule in the right breast
- A 45-year-old woman with 2 weeks of bloody discharge from the left breast

CLINICAL MANIFESTATIONS

The three most common breast symptoms that bring women into the office are lumps, pain, and discharge, in that order. Women may also complain of skin changes such as dimpling, erythema, and nodules.

Women may have no symptoms, or they may have pain or breast nodularity or thickening, soreness or sensitivity, changes in nipple areola or skin, or nipple discharge. The duration and fluctuation of symptoms with the menstrual cycle, and association with lumps or menstrual period are important to the diagnosis.

Pain

Breast pain is common and nonspecific. The most common cause is a cyst or area of fibrocystic changes. The pain may be cyclic or continuous. Cyclic pain suggests hormone-related causes, such as cysts that enlarge with menses.

Pain may be related to a mass, cyst, or thickening. Evaluation should then continue. A mammogram is indicated if the woman is older than 35 years of age; an ultrasound is indicated if the woman is younger than 35 years of age. If the physical examination and mammogram are not suggestive of cancer, the most likely diagnosis is fibrocystic changes with functional menstrual cycle influences.

Nipple Discharge

Nipple discharge can be yellow, bloody (red), pink, multicolored, clear, purulent, or white (Table 3.1). White discharges, especially if bilateral and multiductal, are usually

T ABLE 3.1. Characteristics of nipple discharge

More Suspicious for Cancer	Less Suspicious for Cancer
Bloody, serous, serosanguineous, clear	Gray, black, brown, green, milky
Mass present	No mass present
Unilateral, coming from one duct	Bilateral, multiductal

milk; a patient with such a discharge needs evaluation for galactorrhea. Purulent discharges (i.e., discharges containing pus) indicate an infection, and culture and antibiotics are needed. Yellow or multicolored discharges can suggest ductal ectasia, or lymphatic drainage. This is treated with heat and nonsteroidal anti-inflammatory drugs (NSAIDs). Cancer is rare in patients with this discharge. Clear discharge correlates with ductal carcinoma *in situ*. Between one-third and one-half of these cases are caused by cancer. Pink or bloody discharge is serious and possibly pathologic, and it requires further evaluation. Twenty-five percent of these cases are caused by cancer.

Nipple discharge that is spontaneous is not galactorrhea and is more serious. Nipple discharge that is associated with a lump, unilateral or confined to one duct, is worrisome. Nipple discharge in postmenopausal women is more serious.

There are no good data about the best evaluation of nipple discharge. The discharge may be caused by cancer even with normal mammography, ultrasonography, and cytology. Some studies have stated that cytology is useless. The best evaluation, realizing there are no truly reliable data, is shown in Fig. 3.1.

Lumps/Masses

Any mass in a postmenopausal woman must be considered to be cancer until proved otherwise, even if the patient is taking replacement hormones. Any lump or thickening with an inflammatory appearance in any woman older than 40 years of age should be considered inflammatory Bca until proved otherwise. Biopsy of the breast and skin is indicated.

Cysts

Cysts (Fig. 3.2) are common in premenopausal and postmenopausal women older than 40 years of age. The physical examination cannot always distinguish between cysts and cancer. If a mass is suspected of being a cyst, this can be confirmed rapidly and easily by fine-needle aspiration (FNA). When cysts are aspirated, they should dis-

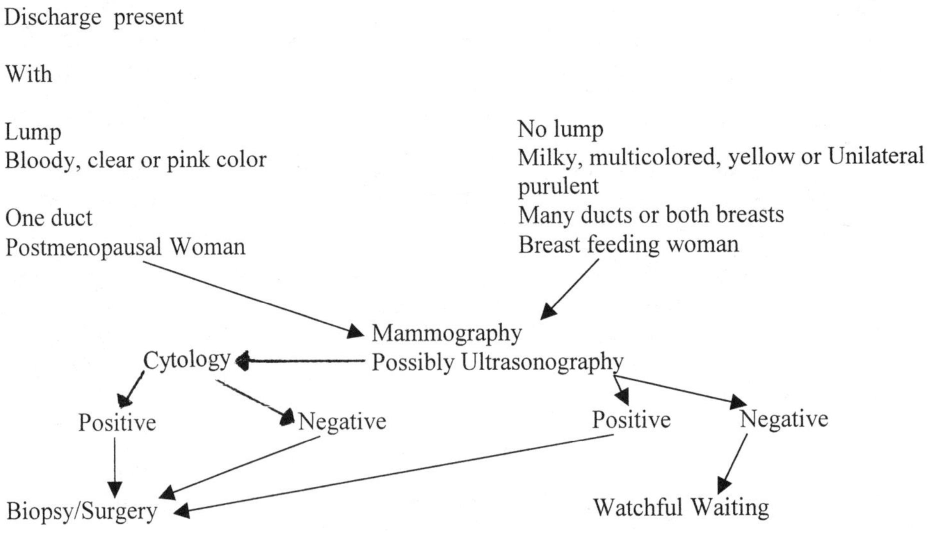

Discharge present

With

Lump	No lump
Bloody, clear or pink color	Milky, multicolored, yellow or Unilateral purulent
One duct	Many ducts or both breasts
Postmenopausal Woman	Breast feeding woman

Mammography
Cytology ◄——— Possibly Ultrasonography

Positive   Negative   Positive   Negative

Biopsy/Surgery   Watchful Waiting

FIGURE 3.1. Evaluation of nipple discharge.

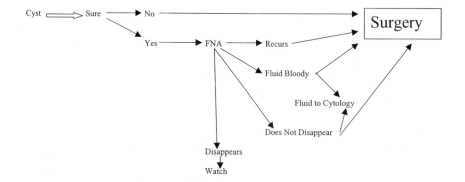

FIGURE 3.2. Evaluation of breast cyst.

appear. If a cyst does not disappear completely or the fluid is bloody, the fluid should be sent for pathologic analysis and the patient should have a biopsy or surgery. A woman with a cyst should be watched for recurrence. If the cyst recurs, surgery or biopsy should be advised.

Solid Masses

A suspicious mass should always be referred to a surgeon, even if the mammogram is negative. An open-excisional surgical biopsy is preferred for a solid mass that is dominant, discrete, and palpable. FNA may be used only as the preliminary diagnostic approach. If the patient feels a mass not felt by the physician and has a normal mammogram, waiting and rechecking are reasonable.

Masses in young women are most likely fibroadenomas because in this age group cancer is rare. FNA or ultrasound may make the diagnosis. However, if the woman has a suspicious, discrete, solitary, or noncystic lesion, biopsy or surgical excision is indicated.

Women with an area of thickening that is read on mammogram as a nonsuspicious mass and cannot be felt by the physician can be observed clinically every 3 to 6 months.

Vague Nodularity

With vague nodularity the woman feels a mass, perhaps during her premenstrual period, but the examiner does not and the mammogram is normal. If the woman is concerned or anxious, have her return bimonthly or every 3 months until it disappears or results continue to be benign. If she was menstruating, have her return at midcycle. If the vague nodularity persists for more than 3 months, consider referral to a surgeon and FNA.

EPIDEMIOLOGY

BCa is the third most frequent cancer in the world and is the most common malignancy in women, causing 21% of all new cases, and the leading cause of cancer mortality in women. In American women it accounts for 32% of malignancies. However, when compared with other cancers, BCa has a high survival rate.

The incidence of BCa increases with age. BCa rates are higher in developed countries.

RISK FACTORS

Risk factors can be seen in Table 3.2.

Age. The incidence of BCa increases with age (Fig. 3.3). However, BCa in the elderly has a relatively slower tumor growth rate.

Family history. Any woman who has a first-degree relative who developed BCa while she was premenopausal has a risk that is three to four times greater than normal of developing BCa. If a woman has a first-degree relative who had bilateral cancer when she was premenopausal or more than one first-degree postmenopausal relative with BCa, her risk of BCa is eight to 10 times that of the general population.

If a woman has several second-degree relatives with BCa, including men, she has an increased risk of BCa, even if her relatives developed the cancer postmenopausally.

Women with a family history of the disease are more likely to have screening mammograms. They chronically have increased worry, and this worry makes them more likely to get screening tests.

Previous history of BCa. Ten percent of women with BCa develop a secondary primary BCa during their lifetimes.

Obstetric history. If a woman is nulliparous or if her first pregnancy occurs after 35 years of age, she has an increased risk of BCa.

Early menarche (before age 12) or **late menopause** (after age 53).

Radiation exposure in the breast area as a child.

History of malignant disease in childhood or adolescence, particularly Hodgkin's disease, that may have led to radiation exposure.

Environmental risk factors, such as pollutants with weakly estrogenic potential (e.g., polychlorinated biphenyls and DDT pesticide), may be the reason for the increased incidence of BCa, although there has not been good evidence to link the exposure and BCa risk in humans.

T ABLE 3.2.   Risk factors for breast cancer

Age
Family history
    Particularly a first-degree relative (mother, sister, aunt) and especially if premenopausal
Previous history of breast cancer
Early menarche (before age 12)
Late menopause (after age 53)
Nulliparity or first child after age 35
Radiation exposure to breast as a child
History of malignant disease during childhood or adolescence (particularly Hodgkin's)
Race

Percent of Women Developing Breast Cancer by Age

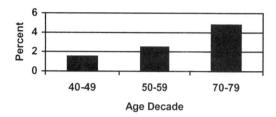

FIGURE 3.3. Percent of women in whom breast cancer develops by age; the risk increases with age.

Race. In African-Americans, BCa is more likely to be present before 40 years of age. Body mass index and obesity are stronger risk factors for BCa in African-Americans. African-American women are more likely to present late and may seek alternative care. They have a poorer survival rate.

Obesity. Women in the highest quartile for body mass index are at higher risk for BCa.

Use of birth control pills. Use of oral contraceptive pills is not a risk for BCa. In fact, it may be protective.

Hormone replacement therapy may increase the risk of developing BCa.

Prevention and Screening for All Women
Women Younger Than 40 Years of Age

1. A clinical breast examination (CBE) should be included in any complete physical examination.
2. Screening mammograms are of debatable value in this age group for asymptomatic women who are not at high risk. The sensitivity of a mammogram is between 61% and 87%; it is lower in women younger than 50 years of age (56%) than in those more than 50 years of age (78%), probably because of increased radiodensity of the premenopausal breast. Mammograms are very effective in identifying most cancers in all age groups but are more sensitive in older women. Mammograms miss 10% of cancers in women under 50 years of age but only 5% of those in women more than 50 years of age. In women under 35 years of age, mammograms are not recommended, and ultrasonography is useful if a diagnostic test is needed. No screening radiologic test is suggested.

Women 40 to 49 Years of Age

1. Annual CBEs are indicated.
2. Annual screening mammograms are indicated in women 40 to 49 years of age. Although there still is conflicting discussion of the benefit of an annual mammogram to decrease mortality for this age group, the American Cancer Society (ACS) and National Cancer Institute (NCI) recommend a mammogram every year for asymptomatic women age 40 and up regardless of risk group. A 1999 consensus

statement in *JAMA* suggests that without risk factors or a family history, annual screening is still not indicated in all women 40 to 49 years of age.

Women 50 to 69 Years of Age

The following are Level A recommendations from the U.S. Preventive Services Task Force:
1. Annual CBEs are indicated.
2. Annual screening mammograms are indicated. A screening mammogram is sensitive; it can detect nonpalpable BCa, both invasive and noninvasive.
3. Self breast examination (SBE) is suggested. Women who perform SBE are more likely to have annual CBEs and mammograms, although the benefit of SBE as a screening tool to reduce mortality has not been proved.

Women Older Than 70 Years of Age

A screening mammogram has not been shown to decrease BCa mortality in women more than 70 years of age. Although a mammogram is more specific and has higher sensitivity in older women because of gradual replacement of glandular breast tissue by fat, screening mammograms are not universally suggested by ACS guidelines.

There is little information about the effects of screening in older women. There have been few women more than 75 years of age in screening studies. Benign lesions are less common in older patients. However, screening women older than 70 years of age may be helpful. In one study, it was estimated that the relative risk of dying from BCa between the ages of 70 and 75 for women who had undergone a recent screening was 38% of that for women who had not been screened. A 1997 ACS consensus statement on screening stated that cessation of annual screening is a function not of age but of comorbidity and that there is no age at which screening should be terminated.

Other Screening Methods

In high-risk groups, magnetic resonance imaging (MRI) may be a tool for the detection of BCa. MRI is more sensitive than mammograms or ultrasound. The combined protocol of clinical examination, mammogram, and FNA has a predictive value for benign disease of 99% when all three are negative. Table 3.3 gives BCa screening recommendations for all women.

TABLE 3.3.   Screening recommendations for breast cancer for every woman

	Age			
	<40	**40–49**	**50–69**	**>70**
Self–breast examination	Suggested	Suggested	Suggested	Suggested
Clinical breast examination	Yes	Yes	Yes	Yes
Mammography yearly	No	Possibly*	Yes	Possibly†

*One screening examination is suggested for everyone. The American Cancer Society has decided on one screening mammography yearly. A 1999 consensus statement in *JAMA* suggests yearly mammography only for women at risk, and perhaps yearly after age 45, but the evidence is still unclear if it decreases mortality for everyone.

†Cessation of yearly mammography is a function of history and comorbidity and not of age alone.

Screening in Women with Risk Factors

Women with risk factors, especially a family history of a first-degree relative (mother, sister, aunt) with BCa, should have an annual mammographic screening along with an annual examination from age 25, and ultrasound as needed. It is especially important for these women to be screened annually if their first-degree relatives developed the cancer before menopause, or if two second-degree relatives have had BCa.

DIAGNOSIS

Examination

Note size, shape, attachment to surrounding tissue and chest wall, presence or absence of other masses or cysts in that and the other breast, and presence or absence of axillary nodes. Note skin above the mass and any changes or attachment.

Masses that are large, solid, hard, fixed to the chest wall, and nonfluctuant and that present with skin changes, nipple retraction, or axillary nodes are more likely to be cancer.

Mammography

Mammographic reports have six categories of abnormalities (Table 3.4). Evaluation of a woman with a solid suspicious mass should include bilateral mammogram and may include ultrasound or aspiration. The primary purpose of the mammogram is to screen normal tissue and the opposite breast for nonpalpable cancers, not to make a diagnosis.

In women under 35 years of age, ultrasonography may be a first choice, although a mammogram should be performed. A normal mammogram at any age does not eliminate the need for further evaluation of a palpable mass.

Ultrasound

Ultrasonography differentiates between solid and cystic masses. If a mass is seen on mammogram, especially in young women, ultrasonography can help differentiate cystic from solid masses. Ultrasound can diagnose a simple cyst. This will show up as round or oval, with sharp margins, a lack of internal echoes, and posterior acoustic enhancement.

T ABLE 3.4. Six categories of mammographic results

No.	Meaning	Action
0	Assessment is incomplete; additional imaging necessary	Complete imaging studies with ultrasound or spot compression or magnification
1	Negative finding	None
2	Benign finding	Clinical follow-up as needed
3	Probable benign finding (maximum 2% risk of cancer)	Short interval follow-up suggested; If no mass, watch or refer if patient requests
4	Suspicious abnormality	Biopsy suggested; refer to surgeon
5	Highly suggestive of malignancy	Refer to surgeon

Other Diagnostic Tests
Doppler Sonography
In the diagnosis of a mass to differentiate benign from malignant, advances in color Doppler sonography may lead to improved sensitivity.

Fine-Needle Aspiration
FNA is useful as an adjunct to the clinical evaluation of a breast lump/cyst. Family physicians can learn and perform this procedure in the office. FNA can diagnose and eliminate a fluid-filled cyst or aspirate tissue for cytologic evaluation of a solid mass. The false-positive rate is negligible, but the false-negative rate is as high as 20%. If a mass persists after aspiration, it should be excised. FNA is very good for evaluation of a cyst diagnosed by examination or ultrasound (Fig. 3.2).

Stereotactic-Guided Breast Biopsy
Stereotactic-guided breast biopsy (STBx), or biopsy needle placement by mammograph, supplements mammography findings, reducing the rate of unnecessary excision biopsies.

Two types of STBx are available: (1) stereotactic cutting-needle biopsy, which gives core tissue for histology, and (2) stereotactic needle aspiration, which provides material for cytology. The rate of use for the latter technique is increasing rapidly and is used regularly in two situations: in a woman with an area of clustered microcalcifications seen on mammogram and considered suspicious, and in a woman with areas that mammographically appear to be at low risk of being cancerous but that have changed since the last mammogram.

STBx can effectively sample suspicious clustered calcifications that have a 20% or greater risk of being cancer. At least half of these are *in situ* cancer. Use of STBx would decrease the number of excisional biopsies by identifying noncancerous tissue.

Open Surgical Biopsy
Open surgical biopsy is the gold standard of pathologic assessment of a breast lesion. It can be performed on palpable or nonpalpable lesions after STBx or mammogram localization.

When conducting a surgical biopsy, the biopsy specimen must be wide enough that those with cancer should have a 1-cm free margin of normal tissue. All biopsy or lumpectomy specimens should produce a single intact tissue specimen. The biopsy should be in a single piece, not in multiple pieces.

T ABLE 3.5.   Women with a breast mass who may need immediate referral to surgeon

1. Woman persistently worried, with negative workup
2. Woman whose breasts are difficult to examine because they are large, dense, or multinodular, or scarred from biopsies, pregnancy, or lactation
3. Any pregnant woman with a suspicious mass
4. Women at high risk of breast cancer, including those with atypia on breast biopsy and those with a family history of breast cancer among premenopausal first-degree relatives or several other relatives

REFERRAL

Some women may need immediate referral to a surgeon (Table 3.5). They include women persistently worried with negative workup; women whose breasts are difficult to examine because they are large, dense, or multinodular, or scarred from biopsies, pregnancy, or lactation; any pregnant woman with a suspicious mass (1 in 200 pregnant or lactating women have BCa); women at high risk of BCa, including those with atypia on breast biopsy; and women with a family history of BCa among first-degree relatives or several relatives.

STAGING

Staging is important to help decide treatment and prognosis. The following methods can be used.

Mammogram. Once cancer is diagnosed, the cancer should be staged. A mammogram may not be the best and may be inaccurate, but it can screen for ipsilateral and contralateral occult cancer.

MRI. MRI is more effective for staging tumor size, and local tumor extent.

TREATMENT
BCa Stages I and II
Surgery with Radiation
The standard treatment has been mastectomy, either radical or modified radical. However, breast-conservation surgery (lumpectomy) with local radiation has become the preferred method of treatment for many. Conservative surgery and radiation have a survival rate comparable to that of mastectomy. Six trials have compared mastectomy with conservative surgery and radiation. In follow-up of up to 18 years, there were no differences in overall or disease-free survival with either treatment. All trials had adjuvant chemotherapy as well.

The survival rate is good with conservative therapy. At 10 years, local recurrence rates with negative margins are 10% or less.

To consider conservative therapy, several medical factors have to be evaluated (Table 3.6). Age is not a contraindication, nor is a comorbid condition. Retractions of skin, nipple, and breast parenchyma are also not contraindications (Table 3.7).

The mammogram may show pathologic conditions that would suggest not using breast-conservation surgery. These include vascular or lymphatic invasion, and presence of an inflammatory infiltrate that increases the risk of BCa recurrence.

- **Histologic type and grade.** Some studies show a higher risk of recurrence and thus less likelihood of cure with conservative surgery and radiation in patients with higher histology grade tumors, presence of tumor necrosis, and/or presence of ductal carcinoma *in situ* (DCIS). DCIS is related to a high risk of BCa recurrence. Twenty percent of women with early-stage BCa who undergo conservative surgery have extensive intraductal components; these women have an increased risk of BCa recurrence. This decreases if the surgeon uses a wide surgical resection and achieves negative margins.
- **Margins of resection.** A woman whose surgery has positive margins of resection has an increased risk of recurrence in extensive intraductal negative tumors. Of women whose surgical specimens showed a diffuse margin involvement, 42% had recurrence, compared with none of those with negative margins.

T ABLE 3.6. Information needed to determine if conservative surgery rather than traditional mastectomy can be safely attempted

1. History
   a. Family history
   b. Previous breast irradiation
   c. Previous connective tissue disease
   d. History of breast implants
   e. Nipple discharge
   f. Last menstrual period (LMP); possibility of pregnancy
2. Physical examination
   a. Tumor size and ratio of breast size to tumor size
   b. Whether tumor is fixed to skin
   c. Evidence of multiple tumors
   d. Axillary and supraclavicular node status
   e. Evidence of locally advanced cancer
3. Mammography
   a. Size, extent
   b. Calcifications
   c. Multicentricity
4. Pathology
   a. Vascular or lymphatic invasion
   b. Histologic type and grade
   c. Absence or presence of tumor necrosis
   d. Presence of ductal carcinoma *in situ*
   e. Presence of an inflammatory infiltrate
   f. Margins of resection
   g. Status of axillary nodes
5. Patient preferences

T ABLE 3.7. Absolute and relative contraindications for conservative breast surgery and radiation

1. Absolute contraindications
   a. Pregnancy
   b. Two or more primary tumors in separate quadrants of the breast
   c. Diffuse malignant-appearing microcalcifications
   d. Previous therapeutic irradiation to the breast region
   e. Persistent positive margins after reasonable surgical attempts
2. Relative contraindications
   a. Collagen vascular disease—scleroderma or lupus
   b. Multiple gross tumors in the same quadrant and indeterminate calcifications
   c. The presence of a large tumor in a small breast
   d. Large breast size

Data from: Winchester DP, Cox JD. Standards for diagnosis and management of invasive breast carcinoma. *CA Cancer J Clin* 1998;48:83.

T ABLE 3.8. Survival rates of women with breast cancer

	Adjusted Survival Rate (%)
Noninvasive cancer	97.2
Invasive cancer	78.2
With negative nodes	85.5
<1 cm	90.2
1–1.9 cm	80.5
2.0–4.9 cm	70.5
>5 cm	60.6

Data from: Smart CR, Byrne C, Smith RA. Twenty-year follow-up of the breast cancers diagnosed during the breast cancer detection demonstration project. *CA Cancer J Clin* 1997;47:134.

- **Axillary node involvement.** Even with positive axillary nodes, women do well with conservative therapy and radiation. However, in women undergoing mastectomy, the number of positive nodes is related to the incidence of chest wall recurrence and survival (Table 3.8).

Adjuvant Therapy

Adjuvant chemotherapy is administered to "downstage" the tumor and enable breast-conserving surgery. Use of adjuvant chemotherapy or tamoxifen (Nolvadex) may reduce the 5-year recurrence rate of BCa in patients with positive margins (see discussion later).

Stage III and Higher

Adjuvant chemotherapy is the treatment of choice for advanced BCa and is used in almost all such cases (Table 3.9).

T ABLE 3.9. Current treatment regimens by disease state

Stages I and II	
Premenopausal lesion	
<1 cm and node negative	Mastectomy or Lumpectomy with chest radiation
1–2 cm	Above plus adjuvant chemotherapy
Stage II and lesion 2–5 cm or node positive	Surgery and adjuvant chemotherapy
	Nodal and/or chest wall radiation
	Tamoxifen for 5 years if estrogen positive
Postmenopausal stage II	Adjuvant chemotherapy and surgery
High risk, receptor-negative tumor	Adjuvant chemotherapy and surgery
Positive nodes	Nodal radiation
Stage III—locally advanced	Adjuvant chemotherapy and surgery
	Surgery, radiotherapy, and chemotherapy

Hormonal Suppression

Approximately 60% to 70% of cancers found positive for estrogen or progesterone receptors respond to hormonal suppression, and a response increases the survival rate. Tamoxifen, an antiestrogen, has been used for more than 20 years. Women with estrogen receptor-positive tumors benefit the most from hormonal suppression, with reduced relapse and mortality rates. Tamoxifen is used in postmenopausal patients and receptor-positive patients with lesions larger than 1 cm. Tamoxifen is also being evaluated as a preventive agent in women at high risk for BCa.

Ovarian oblation has been shown to decrease the recurrence rate and increase overall survival in women with BCa who are younger than 50 years of age.

Cytotoxic Chemotherapy

More than 20 years ago, chemotherapy after modified mastectomy or lumpectomy with radiation was shown to improve survival in premenopausal women with node-positive cancer. Multidrug cytotoxic chemotherapy is now also recommended in node-negative premenopausal and postmenopausal women except for women with negative nodes and lesions less than 1 cm. The most effective combinations are cyclophosphamide (Cytoxan), methotrexate, and 5-fluorouracil (CMF); and cyclophosphamide (Cytoxan), doxorubicin (Adriamycin), and 5-fluorouracil (CAF). The effect of chemotherapy on certain subgroups is under investigation.

Radiotherapy

Radiotherapy provides optimal local and regional disease control in many patients, especially those in stages I and II. Nodal radiation is needed in women with positive nodes and/or lesions between 2 and 5 cm. For locally advanced disease (stage III), nodal and chest wall radiation is used.

FOLLOW-UP

Survival and Recurrence Rates

Survival rates (Table 3.8) of 97% are observed for women with noninvasive cancer, and of 78% for those with invasive cancer. Lymph node status and size of cancer at diagnosis are prognostic indicators of survival. Table 3.10 lists some of the many indicators of poor prognosis or recurrence.

Follow-up care has the following goals:
• Early detection of recurrence or new cancer
• Treatment of sequelae
  Follow-up should include the following:
• **A good history and physical examination.** During the first 3 years, office visits should be scheduled every 3 to 6 months; during the fourth and fifth years, the patient should be seen every 6 months, and annually after the fifth year.
• **Mammogram.** The changes that occur in the first 12 months (e.g., thickening) should be "normal" by 12 months. Do a baseline for comparison at 3 to 9 months, then a mammogram annually.

Genetic Issues

Specific BCA1 and BCA2 genes occur in families in which BCa occurs early and is more common than in the general population. These genes are responsible for hereditary BCas and represent only 0.3% of all BCa patients. In Ashkenazi Jewish women, 1% carry the BRCA1 mutation and 1% the BRCA2 mutation. Other, less frequent gene mutations linked to BCa include p53, ataxia telangiectasis syndrome, and HRAS1, which together are responsible for only 5% to 10% of all hereditary BCas.

T ABLE 3.10. Tumor-related prognostic factors

1. Histologic type
   Ductal carcinoma *in situ* — 98% cure rate
   Invasive carcinoma mucinous, tubular, — 100% cure rate if <1.0 cm
   medullary, and papillary CA — 91% cure rate if 1 < 3.0 cm
2. Age — Women 40–49 had better survival with noninvasive or invasive cancer totally and those <5 cm
3. Anatomic staging
   Metastases to regional lymph nodes — Without adjuvant chemotherapy and without positive nodes, cure rate is only 76%;
   Without adjuvant chemotherapy and with positive nodes, cure rate is 24%;
   With four or more nodes positive, cure rate is 17%
   Number of nodes — 0 nodes positive, 75%
   1–3 nodes positive, 62%
   4–9 nodes positive, 42%
   >9 nodes positive, 20%
4. Tumor size — <1.0 cm, 88% to 96%
5. Steroid hormone receptor proteins — If present, often associated with other favorable indicators; by itself, a weak correlation with more positive outcome
6. Aneuploidy (increased DNA) — Operable tumors that are diploid up to 1.3 cm have a favorable prognosis

Data from Donegan WD. Tumor related prognostic factors for breast cancer. *CA Cancer J Clin* 1997;47:28.

A woman carrying the BRCA1 or BRCA2 gene mutation has a lifetime risk of 56% to 85% of developing BCa.

When a young woman develops BCa, the chance she is a carrier of hereditary cancer is higher; as many as 33% of women under 30 years of age who develop BCa carry BRCA1 or BRCA2.

Genetic testing is appropriate in women who have a positive family history of BCa and who have one first-degree relative who had cancer when younger than 30 years of age in addition to women who have two first-degree relatives or a male relative with BCa and who desire genetic screening. If a patient wants to be screened, her affected relatives need to be screened first. If they are positive, the patient should be tested for mutations.

Follow-up for women who test positive for BRCA1 or BRCA2 should include the following:
- Monthly SBEs from 18 to 24 years of age
- Monthly SBEs and annual clinical breast examinations and mammograms from 25 years of age

Whether prophylactic mastectomy is indicated or should be offered after childbearing years is disputed. With women with BRCA1, additional CA-125 and pelvic ultrasounds to investigate the possibility of ovarian cancer are suggested. Whether prophylactic oophorectomy should be encouraged after 40 years of age is disputed.

CHAPTER 4

···

Menopause

C. Carolyn Thiedke

Menopause is the time in a woman's life in which the menses cease for greater than 12 months. The etiology is the loss of active ovarian follicles with subsequent diminution of the predominant female hormones estriol, estradiol, and progesterone. The sequelae of this decrease in hormone levels are systemic in a woman's body and, potentially, in her psychosocial functioning.

These days, as millions of baby-boomer women are reaching their 40s and 50s, menopause has become the subject of books, articles, TV talk shows, and workshops. This generation of women has been raised with the idea that they are in charge of their health, and they are eager to discuss their options with their physicians.

CHIEF COMPLAINTS

- A 47-year-old woman presents to your office complaining of heavy, irregular periods for the past 6 months.
- A 53-year-old woman presents to your office to discuss hot flashes occurring almost nightly. They are disrupting her sleep, leading to fatigue during the day.
- A 64-year-old woman with hypertension and type 2 diabetes mellitus presents for a yearly examination. She had a hysterectomy and oophorectomy at 46 years of age for uterine leiomyoma.
- A 72-year-old white woman falls on the ice outside her home and fractures her left hip.

CLINICAL MANIFESTATIONS

The effects of the decline of estrogen are protean. Although some conditions, such as dementia and cardiovascular disease, cannot correctly be referred to as estrogen-deficiency conditions, there is mounting evidence that estrogen deficiency may be one major factor among others.

Hot flashes are the perception of heat within the body. These are accompanied by sudden skin flushing, often of the face and upper chest. Many women report rapid heart beat and light-headedness.

Thinning of the vaginal epithelium leads to a foreshortened vagina with a loss of rugal folds. Mucosal epithelium becomes more friable. Dyspareunia becomes a common complaint.

Thinning of the urethra and atrophy of the bladder trigone occur as well. The relationship of these estrogen-related changes to urinary symptoms of dysuria, frequency, stress, and urge incontinence is commonly held but not well established by research.

Thinning of the epidermis and dermis in response to lowered estrogen levels is suggested by animal and cellular studies, but evidence in humans has not been extensively researched. Two large population-based, cross-sectional studies looking at the effect of estrogen on the skin had conflicting results (Bauer, 1999; Dunn, 1997).

Osteoporosis is generally believed to be a disease of estrogen deficiency, although some researchers have found a decline in bone mineral density occurring during perimenopause before there is a significant fall in estrogen levels (Hernandez, Seco-Durban, Revilla, et al., 1995). Although this may be true, loss of estrogen accelerates the rate of bone loss several times over.

Depression is commonly believed, at least by the lay population, to be a frequent concomitant condition of menopause. Multiple studies of different designs have not found an increase in moderate to severe depression during menopause (Hallstrom and Samuelsson, 1985; Holte and Mikkelsen, 1990). Mild symptoms of depression, however, may peak in the perimenopausal years. Studies in women seeing their doctors for menopausal symptoms do show an association between symptomatic menopause and reports of depression (Hunter and Liao, 1995). Women with a history of depression may notice a resurgence of symptoms during these transitional years (Avis, Brambilla, and McKinlay, 1994).

Memory loss is a frequent complaint among patients as they age. Studies of cognitive function using paper-and-pencil tests show improved performance in women taking estrogens (Dallongeville, Marecaux, Isorez, et al., 1995).

Cholesterol levels, levels of apolipoprotein (apo)B, triglycerides, apo A-1, LDL, and diastolic blood pressure have all been found to be higher in postmenopausal women than in premenopausal women (Dallongeville, Marecaux, Isorez, et al., 1995). Levels of low-density lipoproteins (HDL) have been found to be lower (Dallongeville, Marecaux, Isorez, et al., 1995).

EPIDEMIOLOGY

Family history. Women appear to enter menopause at approximately the same time that their mothers did.

Age. The median age at menopause is 51, with a range of 35 to 58 years.

Culture. Perceptions of menopause vary from culture to culture. Japanese, Indonesian, and Mayan women report low rates of menopausal symptoms (0 to 10%) compared with women from Western cultures (Beyene, 1986; Lock, Kaufert, Gilbert, 1998). In U.S. studies the prevalence of hot flashes ranged from 50% to 85% (Guide to Clinical Preventive Services, 1996).

RISK FACTORS

All women go through menopause if they live long enough. However, several factors appear to affect the age of menopause:
- **Cigarette smoking** has been found to be a consistent link with earlier onset of menopause.
- **Cancer chemotherapy** induces early menopause.
- **Early age of menarche** is associated with later age of menopause, as is higher parity.
- **Menstrual cycles shorter than 26 days** are associated with earlier menopause.
- **Gynecologic surgery,** particularly hysterectomy without oophorectomy, may lead to early menopause.

PATHOLOGY

The transition from perimenopause into menopause is marked by a dwindling number of maturing ovarian follicles. More and more cycles become anovulatory. In general, follicle-stimulating hormone (FSH) levels begin to rise, but estrogen levels may fluctuate widely. By late perimenopause, follicles no longer ovulate under the influence of gonadotrophins. The ovary shifts from a follicle-rich producer of estrogen and progesterone to a stromal-rich producer of androgens. Estrone and estradiol are produced largely by the peripheral aromatization of androstenedione and testosterone. A small amount of progesterone is produced by the adrenal gland.

DIAGNOSIS

Menopause is generally a diagnosis based on history. Confusion may arise, however, during the perimenopausal period when women are beginning to experience single symptoms such as irregular periods, menorrhagia (heavy bleeding), and other symptoms such as hot flashes, irritability, or mood swings. It may be unclear whether menopause might be imminent or whether these symptoms represent some other problem, such as leiomyomata or a mood disturbance.

Serum FSH levels have often been used as a determinant of menopausal status, but the variability of hormone levels in women in their 40s, even in those who continue to have regular cycles, make FSH an undependable indicator. Inhibin A and B, two hormones secreted by the ovaries, are more direct measures of ovarian function but assays are not widely available.

REFERRAL

Because of their broad range of training, family physicians are ideally suited to guide a woman through menopause. Discussions about risk factors, family history, lifestyle changes, and treatment options for menopausal symptoms, heart disease, and osteoporosis are the natural purview for family physicians and their female patients. Perimenopausal menorrhagia, not controlled by hormonal therapy, may require referral to a gynecologist. Postmenopausal bleeding can be initially evaluated by a family physician by vaginal ultrasonography and/or endometrial biopsy but will require referral if those tests are suspicious for cancer.

MANAGEMENT

Estrogen Replacement

In most cases, estrogen replacement quickly relieves hot flashes, the symptom that most often brings patients into the physician's office for treatment. There is convincing evidence that estrogen retards bone loss, favorably affects lipid profiles, and improves cognition. Well-designed randomized controlled clinical trials are lacking, however. The Women's Health Initiative (WHI) currently under way will answer many of these important questions. Results are expected in 2005. It is important for women to understand the many benefits of estrogen replacement therapy (Table 4.1, Fig. 4.1).

The Guide to Clinical Preventive Services, 2nd edition, issued by the U.S. Preventive Services Task Force, makes the following statement regarding postmenopausal hormone prophylaxis: "There is insufficient evidence to recommend for or against hormonal therapy for all postmenopausal women. Women should participate fully in the decision-making process, and individual decisions should be based on patient risk factors for disease, clear understanding of the probable benefits and risks of hormonal therapy, and personal patient preferences."

This is a very complex issue for both physicians and patients. Two books, both written in recent years by women physicians for the lay public, contain self-assessment questionnaires that can be used to guide a woman through this important decision (Col, 1997; Love, 1997).

T ABLE 4.1. Conditions that appear to benefit from hormone replacement therapy

Hot flashes, night sweats
Vaginal dryness
Sexual functioning
Libido
Serum lipids
Urinary incontinence
Recurrent urinary tract infections
Cognitive functioning
Mood
Osteoporosis
Risk of coronary heart disease
Risk of colon cancer
Quality of life in rheumatoid arthritis
Loss of dentition
Macular degeneration

Estrogen

Estrogens are available in many forms. Conjugated equine estrogens, taken orally, are the most widely used. A synthetic conjugated estrogen that is not equine in origin has now been approved by the Food and Drug Administration. Plant-based estrogens in the form of estradiol or estropipate are also commonly used in oral form. Esterified estrogens are approved for the treatment of vasomotor instability, but there are no data on bone mineral density.

Transdermal estrogens have been available for several years and represent a real advantage for women with liver disease. These relieve menopausal symptoms and have a favorable impact on bone, but because they escape the first-pass liver effect, they do not possess the favorable affect on lipids seen with oral forms. Estrogen creams are also available for the treatment of vaginal dryness. They have also been used in the treatment of urinary incontinence and recurrent urinary tract infections in the elderly. Other products include a ring containing a slow-release estrogen that is placed intravaginally. The estrogen is released over a 3-month period. This must be used with a progestin.

Progestin

Because of the risk of endometrial cancer, most women with an intact uterus should receive a progestin as well as estrogen. Women who are reluctant to take a progestin because of side effects should be monitored yearly with endometrial sampling. It should be documented in the medical record that the patient made this decision after hearing the risks.

Progesterone is a hormone secreted by the female body. However, it is inactivated when taken orally. Therefore progestins, synthetically produced progesterone, have traditionally been used, most commonly medroxyprogesterone acetate (MPA) or Provera.

Progesterone has been available from compounding pharmacists as a vaginal suppository, a cream, or a micronized oral form that survives breakdown in the stomach. These forms of "natural progesterone" are popular with women who are interested in an alternative to synthetic hormones.

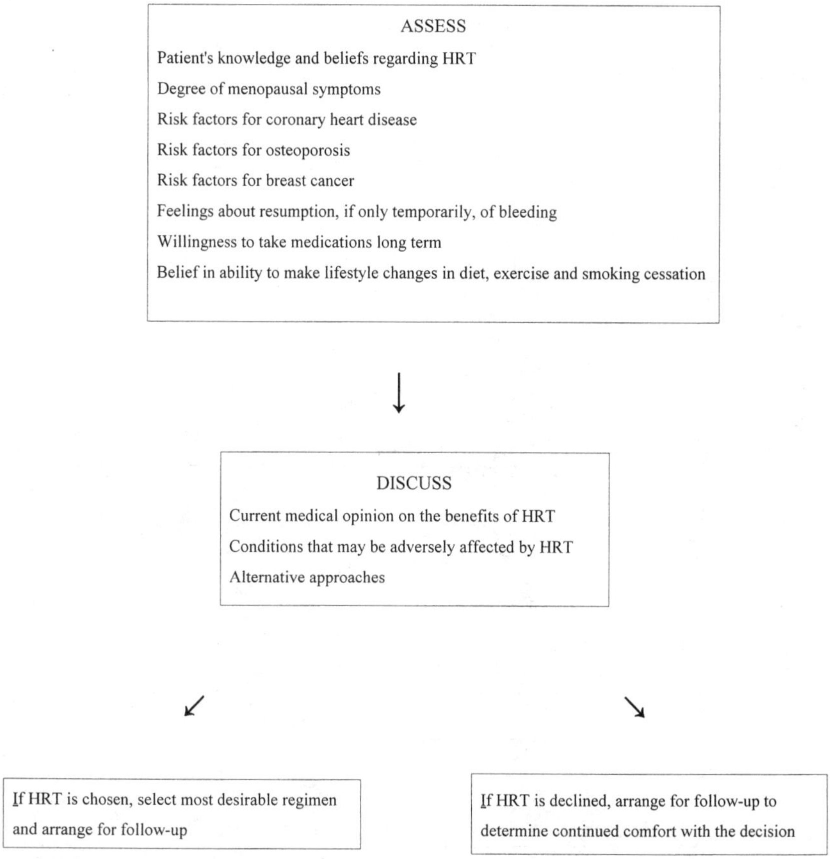

ASSESS

Patient's knowledge and beliefs regarding HRT

Degree of menopausal symptoms

Risk factors for coronary heart disease

Risk factors for osteoporosis

Risk factors for breast cancer

Feelings about resumption, if only temporarily, of bleeding

Willingness to take medications long term

Belief in ability to make lifestyle changes in diet, exercise and smoking cessation

↓

DISCUSS

Current medical opinion on the benefits of HRT

Conditions that may be adversely affected by HRT

Alternative approaches

If HRT is chosen, select most desirable regimen and arrange for follow-up

If HRT is declined, arrange for follow-up to determine continued comfort with the decision

FIGURE 4.1. Model for collaborating with the patient to decide whether hormone replacement therapy (HRT) is appropriate.

Recently, a pharmaceutical company has released a micronized progesterone product (Prometrium) making it more widely available. In the Postmenopausal Estrogen/Progestin Intervention (PEPI) study, women who took estrogen alone or estrogen plus micronized progesterone had a more favorable lipid profile than those who took estrogen plus the synthetic progestin MPA (Table 4.2).

Regimen

Women taking estrogen plus a progestin have traditionally taken them in cyclic fashion in an attempt to mimic physiologic hormone fluctuations. Recent studies have shown that taking both estrogen and progestin continuously affords the same benefits for menopausal symptoms and osteoporosis prevention, without causing the resumption of cyclic bleeding that women find troubling. There is interest in a regimen where the progestin is taken every third month to promote sloughing of the endometrium, but studies are not yet available (Table 4.3).

T ABLE 4.2. Preparations of progestins for HRT*

Brand Name	Generic Name	Dose in Hormone Replacement Therapy	Comment
Provera/	Medroxyprogesterone	5–10 mg	Cyclic dose
Cycrin/Amen	acetate (MPA)	2.5–5 mg	Daily dose
Micronor	Norethindrone	0.15 mg	Cyclic dose
Prometrium	Micronized progesterone	200–300 mg	Cyclic dose

*Not approved by the U.S. Food and Drug Administration for this use.

T ABLE 4.3. Hormone replacement therapy regimen options

Hormone	Schedule of Estrogen	Schedule of Progesterone	Comment
Estrogen only	Daily	None	For women who have had a hysterectomy or those monitored yearly
Cyclic	Daily	10 days of the month	Traditional method, monthly bleeding
Continuous combined	Daily	Daily	Lower-dose progestin, menses will stop in most women
Every-3-months progesterone	Daily	14 days every 3 months	Newer data

T ABLE 4.4. Preparations of combination products for HRT

Brand Name	Generic Name	Dose	Comment
Prempro	CEE/MPA	0.625 mg/2.5 mg	Continuous regimen
Premphase	CEE/MPA	0.625 mg/5 mg	Cyclic regimen
Combipatch	Estradiol/Norethindrone acetate	0.05 mg/0.14 mg 0.05 mg/0.25 mg	Changed twice per week
Alesse*	Ethinyl estradiol/ Levongestrol	20 mcg/0.1 mg	For perimenopausal menorrhagia
Mircette*	Ethinyl estradiol/ Desogestrel	50 mcg/0.15 mg	For perimenopausal menorrhagia
Loestrin*	Ethinyl estradiol/ Norethindrone acetate	30 mcg/1.5 mg	For perimenopausal menorrhagia
Estratest	Esterified estrogen/ Methyltestosterone	1.25 mg/2.55 mg	Improvement of libido; concerns about virilization and lipids
Estratest H.S.		0.625 mg/1.5 mg	

Abbreviations: CEE, conjugated equine estrogens; MPA, medroxyprogesterone acetate.
*Not approved for this use by the U.S. Food and Drug Administration.

Combination Products

Two pills and a transdermal patch are now available that combine estrogen and MPA. One oral form creates a cyclic regimen and the other, continuous. The transdermal patch creates a continuous regimen. For perimenopausal women with dysfunctional uterine bleeding and the need for contraception, low-estrogen oral contraceptives, such as Alesse or Mircette, can be used. With increasing frequency, physicians are prescribing an estrogen/testosterone combination for women. Placebo-controlled trials have shown beneficial effects on mood and libido when the combination is used (Sherwin, 1999). Concerns arise, however, about the risk of virilization and the adverse effects of androgens on lipid profiles. Acne and hirsutism were noted in two studies (Hickok, Toomey, Speroff, 1993; Watts N, Notelovitz M, Timmons M, et al., 1995), but another randomized, double-blind study showed no increase in hirsutism in women receiving the estrogen/testosterone combination compared with estrogen alone (Phillips and Bainum, 1997). Several studies have shown a drop in HDL when using combination therapy, but it is unclear whether this would reverse the favorable impact of estrogen in coronary atherosclerosis (Table 4.4) (Hickok, Toomey, Speroff, 1993).

T ABLE 4.5.   Estrogen effect on certain conditions: traditional vs. current opinion

Condition	Traditional Opinion	Current Opinion
Breast cancer	Contraindicated	There may be a place for HRT; some data suggest improved quality of life
Endometrial cancer	Contraindicated	Women with treated stage I tumors can use HRT
Malignant melanoma	Contraindicated	No evidence that HRT affects prognosis
Venous thrombosis	Contraindicated	Current users of HRT have two- to threefold increased risk; risk still low at 30/100,000 cases
Hypertension and stroke	Questionable increased risk	No association between HRT and HTN or CVA
Active liver disease	Oral estrogen contraindicated	Transdermal products can be used safely
Hypertriglyceridemia	Avoid, since triglyceride levels may be increased	Monitor and if triglyceride levels increase, switch to transdermal
Uterine leiomyoma	Avoid, since estrogen may increase size	The only randomized trial showed no increase. Women with submucous leiomyoma may have abnormal bleeding requiring ultrasound.
Migraines	Avoid	Trial with HRT. If headaches worsen, switch to estradiol derivative.
Smoking	Concern over increased risk of CHD	No increased risk shown
Gallbladder disease	Concern over increased risk with HRT	There is a twofold increased risk, but this is a treatable condition without excess mortality
Systemic lupus erythematosus	Concern over increased risk with HRT	Nurses Health Study showed twofold increased risk, but still small

Abbreviations: CHD, coronary heart disease; CVA, cerebrovascular accident; HRT, hormone replacement therapy; HTN, hypertension.

Contraindications to Estrogen Therapy

• Unexplained vaginal bleeding
• A history of breast cancer

Extended use of estrogens (longer than 7 to 10 years) has been linked to increased risk of breast cancer in two cohort studies in Europe (Hunt, Vessey, McPherson, 1987; Schairer, Lubin, Troisi, et al., 2000) and one in the United States (Colditz, Hankinson, Hunter, et al., 1995). This prohibition is not universally held, however. There are some who note improved quality of life in breast cancer patients receiving hormone replacement therapy (HRT) (Brewster, DiSaia, Grosen, et al., 1999). This is an enormously important issue that has not been adequately addressed by current research and awaits clarity from the results of the WHI.

Historically, women with migraine headaches, a history of thromboembolism, and liver disease have been considered poor candidates for HRT, but this belief is being challenged (Table 4.5).

FOLLOW-UP

Compliance

Only 30% of women who leave their physician's office with a prescription for HRT are taking it a year later. This may reflect ambivalence about long-term commitment to a medication when one is otherwise feeling well. Many are also concerned about the increased risk of breast cancer associated with estrogen replacement that continues for more than 10 years. It seems clear that women who are most symptomatic are the ones most likely to continue to take HRT (Hunter, O'Dea, Britten, 1997).

Physicians may be able to increase the percentage of women who take HRT by the following:

• Acknowledging the complexity of the issue
• Taking the time to explore a patient's misgivings
• Remaining flexible in discussing options, traditional and alternative
• Indicating a willingness to reevaluate the decision if problems arise

Monitoring Effects of Treatment

Seeing women every 2 to 3 months at the outset of treatment will allow the physician to address areas of uncertainty as they arise and to survey for the presence of troubling side effects. Once a woman is well established on a regimen, yearly examinations are sufficient.

Potential Problems and Complications

Women should be counseled to report unexplained vaginal bleeding immediately. Changes to a lower dose of estrogen or progestin, to a different regimen (cyclic versus continuous), or to a different formulation (synthetic versus natural) may circumvent troubling breast tenderness, bloating, bleeding, or other unwanted side effects.

Alternative Treatments

Many women are reluctant to use a traditional hormone replacement regimen whether from concern about breast cancer or from an uneasiness about using synthetic hormones. For some women, using natural hormones is an acceptable alternative. A natural estrogen is one that is plant-based rather than equine-based. A natural progesterone is also plant-based rather than synthetic.

Other women are not comfortable with hormones in any form. For these women, some alternatives include the following. For **vaginal atrophy and dryness,** only estrogen will replace thinning mucosa. There are over-the-counter products, however, that can act as vaginal lubricants. These include Astroglide, Lubrin, Replens, K-Y jelly, Gyne-Moistrin, and Moist Again.

For **hot flashes,** clonidine (Catapres), in doses of 0.1 to 0.4 mg daily, has been shown to be more efficacious than placebo. Bellargal-S, a combination of phenobarbital, ergotamine tartrate, and the levorotatory alkaloid of belladonna, has also been shown to be helpful, but effects are short-lived, and there are many contraindications. A small placebo-controlled trial demonstrated relief from hot flashes with propranolol (Inderal), but the rate of side effects was significant. There is anecdotal evidence about the effects of vitamins B, C, and particularly E in the relief of hot flashes. The effects are thought to be due to their role as antioxidants. Herbal remedies, such as dong quai and black cohosh, have been popular as alternatives to estrogen therapy, but reports are again largely anecdotal.

Lifestyle changes may be helpful. The practice of wearing more "breathable" clothing such as cotton and layering clothing so pieces can be easily removed is helpful. Keeping the ambient temperature of rooms lower is helpful, as is avoidance of hot or spicy foods, caffeine, and alcohol. Small studies have suggested regular physical activity lessens the frequency of hot flashes. Phytoestrogens, found predominantly in foods containing soy, decrease hot flashes. There is also evidence that soy may have beneficial effects on lipids and bone density. Other studies have shown that women who practiced relaxation regularly had fewer hot flashes. Other women were taught "paced breathing," a biofeedback technique to reduce the frequency of hot flashes.

Patient Education
Grappling with Aging
Much has been written in the past decade by lay authors encouraging women to reframe menopause. It should not be seen as a time of decline but as a period when accumulated life experience, coupled with the easing of traditional social roles for women as wives and mothers, can mean a blossoming of self-expression. Cross-cultural studies have confirmed that in many cultures, menopausal women become liberated from previous constraints and are valued for their wisdom and forthrightness.

Lifestyle Changes
Physicians can encourage reassessment of menopause and help a woman to see that after years of looking after others, it is now time to devote more attention to her own healthy behaviors. Certainly, lifestyle changes in the form of improved diet, regular exercise, smoking cessation, and stress reduction techniques can obviate some of the chronic diseases that occur after menopause.

Making the Decision About HRT
The decision about HRT deserves adequate time to assess the many patient-related factors involved, such as risk factors, family history, and health practices, and to discuss current medical knowledge and options. This may be more than the physician and patient want to tackle in one office visit. Often giving the woman information to read between visits can decrease the information that the physician needs to give face to face, and gives the woman a chance to reflect on her options in her own time. Physicians may want to accumulate articles or books that they can recommend as reading (Table 4.6).

Length of Treatment
Women who receive estrogen should be told that the benefits of estrogen replacement accrue over a long period and that current recommendations are that women take it indefinitely. There are those, however, concerned about the risk of breast cancer with use longer than 5 to 10 years who propose that after 7 to 10 years on estro-

T ABLE 4.6. Selected Estrogen replacement products

Active Ingredient(s)	Brand Name	Dosage Form and Route	Strengths	Min. Daily Estrogen Dose to Prevent Bone Loss*	HRT Indications†
17β-estradiol	Estrace micronized	Oral tablet	0.5, 1, 2 mg	2 mg (po)	V,A,O
	Estrace	Vaginal cream	0.01%	—	A
	Estraderm	Transdermal (twice weekly)	0.05, 0.1 mg/day	0.05 mg/day	V,A,O
	Vivelle		0.0375, 0.05, 0.075, 0.1 mg/day		V,A
	Climara	Transdermal (once weekly)	0.05, 0.075, 0.1mg/day	0.025 mg/day	V,A,O
	Estring	Vaginal ring	2 mg (90-day slow release)	—	A
Estradiol valerate	Delestrogen	Intramuscular	10, 20, 40 mg/mL	—	V,A
Estradiol cypionate	Depo-Estradiol	Intramuscular	5 mg/mL	—	V
Esterified estrogen (mixture of sodium salts of estrogenic substances, primarily estrone)	Estratab	Oral tablet	0.3, 0.625, 1.25, 2.5 mg	0.3 mg	V,A,O
	Menest	Oral tablet	0.3, 0.625, 1.25, 2.5 mg	—	V,A
	Estratest H.S.	Oral tablet	0.625 mg + 1.25 mg methyltestosterone	—	V
	Estratest (Solvay)	Oral tablet	1.25 mg + 2.5 mg methyltestosterone	—	V
Estrone	Kestrones	Intramuscular	5 mg/mL	—	V,A

Estropipate (piperazine estrone sulfate)	Ortho-Est; Ogent	Oral tablet	0.625, 1.25, 2.5, 5 mg	1.25 mg	V,A,O
		Vaginal cream	1.5 mg/g	—	A
Mixture of at least 10 different estrogenic substances primarily derived from urine of pregnant mares	Premarin	Oral tablet	0.3, 0.625, 0.9, 1.25, 2.5 mg	0.625 mg	V,A,O
		Vaginal cream	0.625 mg/g	—	A
		Parenteral injection	25 mg/mL	—	Not indicated for HRT
	Prempro	Combination with progestin	0.625 mg CEE + 2.5 mg medroxyprogesterone acetate	0.625 mg	V,A,O
	Premphase	Combination with progestin	0.625 mg CEE + 5 mg medroxyprogesterone acetate for last 14 days of pack	0.625 mg	V,A,O
Plant-derived synthetic mixture of nine estrogenic components	Cenestin	Oral tablet	0.625, 0.9 mg	—	V

Abbreviations: A, atrophic conditions; CEE, conjugated equine estrogens; HRT, hormone replacement therapy; O, osteoporosis intervention; V, vasomotor symptoms.

*Minimum effective dose for prevention of osteoporosis may be less if elemental calcium intake is high (1,500 mg or more).

†The addition of progesterone therapy for 12–14 days of each month is recommended to reduce the incidence of endometrial cancer in women with a uterus.

gen, women might be switched to another medication, such as alendronate (Fosamax), which would provide continued protection of bone mass or a selective estrogen receptor modulator (SERM) such as raloxifene (Evista) that would provide continued protection of bone mass and lipid effects as well.

Interventions that deal with specific chronic conditions such as heart disease, osteoporosis, sexuality in aging women, and depression will be dealt with in subsequent chapters.

SUGGESTED READINGS

Avis NE, Brambilla D, McKinlay SM, et al. A longitudinal analysis of the association between menopause and depression: results from the Massachusetts Women's Health Study. *Ann Epidemiol* 1994;4:214.

Bauer DC, Grady D, Pressman A, et al. The Study of Osteoporotic Fractures Research Group: skin thickness, estrogen use, and bone mass in older women. *Menopause* 1994;1:131.

Beyene Y. Cultural significance and physiological manifestations of menopause: a biocultural analysis. *Cult Med Psychiatry* 1986;10:47.

Brewster WR, DiSaia PJ, Grosen EA, et al. An experience with estrogen replacement therapy in breast cancer survivors. *Int J Fertil Womens Med* 1999;44:186.

Col N. *A woman doctor's guide to hormone therapy.* Worcester, MA: Tatnuck Bookseller Press, 1997.

Colditz GA, Hankinson SE, Hunter DJ, et al. The use of estrogens and progestins and the risk of breast cancer in postmenopausal women. *N Engl J Med* 1995;332:1589.

Dallongeville J, Marecaux N, Isorez D, et al. Multiple coronary heart disease risk factors are associated with menopause and influenced by substitutive hormonal therapy in a cohort of French women. *Atherosclerosis* 1995;118:123.

Dunn LB, Damesyn M, Moore AA, et al. Does estrogen prevent skin aging? Results from the first National Health and Nutrition Examination Survey (NHANES I). *Arch Dermatol* 1997;133:339.

Guide to Clinical Preventive Services: Report of the U.S. Preventive Services Task Force, 2nd ed. Baltimore: Williams & Wilkins, 1996.

Hallstrom T, Samuelsson S. Mental health in the climacteric: the longitudinal study of women in Gothenburg. *Acta Obstet Gynecol Scand* 1985;64:393.

Hernandez ER, Seco-Durban C, Revilla M, et al. Evaluation of bone density with peripheral quantitative computed tomography in healthy premenopausal, perimenopausal, and postmenopausal women. *Age and Ageing* 1995;24:447.

Hickok L, Toomey C, Speroff L. A comparison of esterified estrogens with and without methyltestosterone: effects on endometrial biopsy and serum lipoproteins in postmenopausal women. *Obstet Gynecol* 1993;82:919.

Holte A, Mikkelsen A. Psychosocial determinants of climacteric complaints. *Maturitas* 1990;12:299.

Hunt K, Vessey M, McPherson K, et al. Long-term surveillance of mortality and cancer incidence in women receiving hormone replacement therapy. *Br J Obstet Gynaecol* 1987;94:620.

Hunter MS, Liao KL. A psychological analysis of menopausal hot flashes. *Br J Clin Psychol* 1995;34:589.

Hunter MS, O'Dea I, Britten N. Decision-making and hormone replacement: a qualitative analysis. *Soc Sci Med* 1997;45:1541.

Lock M, Kaufert P, Gilbert P. Cultural construction of the menopausal syndrome: the Japanese case. *Maturitas* 1998;8:189.

Love S. *Dr. Susan Love's hormone book.* New York: Random House, 1997.

McKinlay SM, Brambilla PJ, Posner JG. The normal menopause transition. *Maturitas* 1992;14:103.

Ottosson UB, Johansson BG, von Schuoultz. Subfractions of high density lipoprotein cholesterol during estrogen replacement therapy: a comparison between progestogens and natural progesterone. *Am J Obstet Gynecol* 1993;151:746.

Phillips E, Bainum C. Safety surveillance of esterified estrogens and methyltestosterone (Estratest and Estratest HS) replacement therapy in the United States. *Clin Ther* 1997;19:1070.

Schairer C, Lubin J, Troisi R, et al. Menopausal estrogen and estrogen-progestin replacement therapy and breast cancer risk. *JAMA* 2000;283:485.

Sherwin BB. Affective changes with menopause and androgen replacement therapy in surgically menopause women. *J Affect Disord* 1988;14:177.

Sherwin BB. Estrogen and cognitive function in women. *Proc Soc Exper Bio Med* 1998;217:1.

Watts N, Notelovitz M, Timmons M, et al. Comparison of oral estrogens and estrogens plus androgen on bone mineral density, menopausal symptoms, and lipid-lipoprotein profiles in surgical menopause. *Obstet Gynecol* 1995;85:529.

CHAPTER 5

Heart Disease

Jo Ann Rosenfeld

Heart disease is the greatest cause of mortality in women. Yet until recently, its impact on women was not well reported and its significance and rate of mortality were underrated and undervalued. Research into coronary heart disease (CHD) has often excluded women. Women, and physicians themselves, have discounted the importance of heart disease. Diagnosis of women with CHD has often been ignored, and diagnostic testing has been denied or postponed. Until recently, treatment of women with CHD has been based on studies done primarily in white men.

CHIEF COMPLAINTS

- A 55-year-old diabetic woman with new onset of pain on exertion
- A 66-year-old woman with sudden onset of shortness of breath
- A 78-year-old woman with sudden confusion

CLINICAL MANIFESTATIONS

The typical presentation of CHD is angina, chest pain in midchest (often described as "crushing") that lasts minutes and is brought on by exertion and relieved by rest. The typical pain of a myocardial infarction (MI) starts as angina, lasts hours, may radiate to the neck or arms, and can be associated with nausea, weakness, palpitations, syncope, diaphoresis, and vomiting.

The clinical presentation of CHD is different in women. The appearance of angina and CHD occurs an average of 10 to 20 years later than that in men. Women are more likely to have angina, whereas men are more likely to have infarction and sudden death as presenting signs of CHD. Women are more likely to have silent MIs than are men. However, as women age, they are more likely to present with symptoms of an acute painful MI.

The symptoms of CHD in women may be different too. In women the pain may be more likely centered in the chest with or without radiation to the ear, jaw, neck, back, or shoulder. Women are more likely to have neck and shoulder pain, nausea, vomiting, fatigue, or dyspnea with chest pain. Women with symptoms tend to delay longer than men before seeking treatment. Women with chronic stable angina are more likely than men to have chest pain during rest, sleep, or periods of mental stress.

Despite identical symptoms or even symptoms that may seem more mild, when a woman presents with CHD, the consequences are often more serious. Women have a higher prevalence of complications after MI, including stroke and cardiac rupture. Women are more likely to die in the hospital after an acute MI.

Physicians react differently when women present with chest pain than when men present. More women visit physicians' offices than men, and women are thought to bring their complaints to their physicians more often. On the other hand, some physicians believe that women complain more and that new complaints are more likely to include an emotional component; thus physicians may take such complaints less seriously than if they were made by men. Women with an exaggerated emotional style are often perceived as having a far lower likelihood of CHD than women with identical histories but a business-like manner.

EPIDEMIOLOGY

CHD is the number-one killer of women older than 50 years of age. More than half a million women die yearly of CHD. The rate of mortality from CHD has decreased in the United States since 1960, with an approximately 2% decrease in mortality rates yearly. In certain groups, however, mortality rates from CHD have not decreased as rapidly. African-American women have mortality rates from CHD that are twice those of white women, making CHD the leading cause of death in African-American women 30 to 39 years of age or older than 65 years of age (Fig. 5.1). African-American women have rates of CHD morbidity that are similar to those white women, but they have higher rates of mortality. This fact is based not on genetics but on socioeconomic factors, including access issues (Table 5.1). The differences in mortality rates between African-American and white women are less for women older than 65 years of age, because the mortality rate in white women increases after age 65.

RISK FACTORS

Being a Woman

Being a woman decreases the risk of CHD until 75 years of age or older. The male-to-female ratio of CHD morbidity is 7:1 in the third decade. This ratio decreases until age 70, when it is equal. Women have MIs at an average age of 75, 10 years later than men.

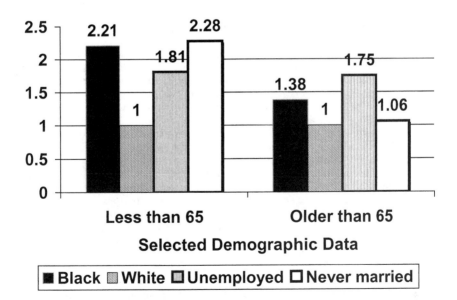

FIGURE 5.1. The effect of factors on risk of heart disease deaths in women. Relative risk of heart dissease mortality (right) according to age (bottom).

T ABLE 5.1.   Relative risk for coronary heart disease in women and men by race

Risk Factor	African-American Women	White Women	African-American Men	White Men
Systolic blood pressure	1.5*	1.55	2.09	1.45
Smoking	1.47*	1.54	0.89	1.49
Serum cholesterol	1.12	1.11	1.47*	1.40

Data taken from Gillium RF, Mussolino ME, Madasn JH. Coronary heart disease risk factors and attributable risks in African American women and men: NHANES I epidemiology followup study. *Am J Public Health* 1998;88:913.
*$p < .05$

Employment

When women started entering the workforce in greater numbers, it was thought that they would get "men's diseases," such as CHD, in greater numbers. Employment was supposed to increase the rate of CHD in women. However, working outside the home by itself does not increase the risk of CHD.

Psychosocial Factors

Psychosocial risk factors for CHD have been studied more in men than in women.
The archetypal type A behavior classification was developed based on upper-middle-class men, and its significance for women of all socioeconomic levels is disputed. Women who have more social support and strong ties to their communities had a decreased total death rate from CHD (Fig. 5.1). The relative risk of death from CHD in an individual with depression or feelings of hopelessness was 1.6 in men and 2.6 in women (Fig. 5.2).

Body Mass Index

Body mass index (BMI) is related to CHD mortality in women and men younger than 65 years of age. BMI does not relate to overall mortality of all causes in women. A BMI greater than 27, or in the highest quartile, increased the risk of CHD deaths (Fig. 5.3).

Obesity

Obesity is an independent risk factor for CHD. Women in the highest category of obesity had a threefold greater risk of CHD than those in the lowest category. Those who were mildly to moderately overweight had two times the risk.
Central obesity is more associated with risk of CHD than is simple body mass. Obesity worsens the risk of several other CHD risk factors, including diabetes, hypertension, and hypercholesterolemia. There was no evidence that losing weight reduces risk of CHD.

Family History

A family history of premature CHD is an independent predictor of risk in women. There is suggestive evidence that, for women as for men, a history of an early MI in either parent (before 60 years of age) increases the risk of CHD in women 2.8 times (relative risk).

Smoking

Smoking is the leading avoidable cause of all deaths in the United States for both men and women. Smoking among American women declined from 34% in 1965 to 23% in

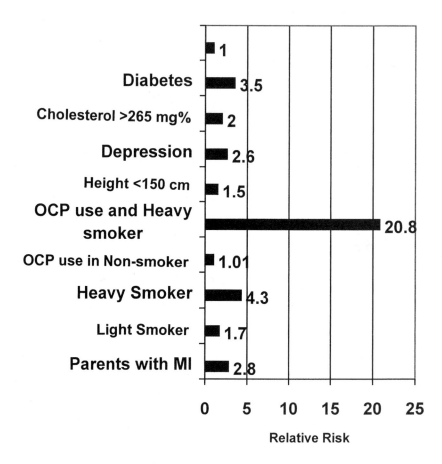

FIGURE 5.2. Relative risk of mortality in women by risk factor. OCP, oral contraceptive pills; MI, myocardial infarction.

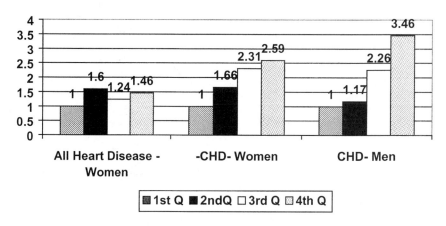

FIGURE 5.3. Relative risk of mortality in white women by BMI. (Data from Dorn JM, Schisterman EF, Winkelstein W, Trevisan M. Body mass index and mortality in a general population sample of men and women: The Buffalo Health Study. *Am J Epidemiol* 1997;146:919.)

1991, but the rate of smoking cessation was lower among women than men. Cigarette smoking increases the risk of MI in women who are light smokers (relative risk, 1.7) and increases it even more in heavy smokers (relative risk, 4.3) (Fig. 5.2). The number of cigarettes smoked daily correlated directly with the risk of MI and fatal CHD. Stopping for 3 years decreased the risk to the level of someone who has never smoked.

Smoking negates the estrogen-induced advantage of decreased CHD risk seen in nonsmoking premenopausal women.

Lipids

Each 1% decrease in cholesterol level has been associated with a 2% to 3% decrease in CHD in men. In women the effects of lipids on CHD and the effects of decreasing lipid levels are less well studied and more complex.

Low-density lipoprotein (LDL) cholesterol elevation is a risk factor for CHD. Low HDL cholesterol is a stronger risk factor for women than for men. Triglyceride elevation increases the risk of CHD. Reducing total cholesterol and LDL cholesterol and increasing HDL-cholesterol will decrease the risk of CHD.

Hypertension

As with men, hypertension is a risk factor for CHD in women. The incidence of hypertension increases with age, just like CHD. However, more women have hypertension than men because women live longer. Eighty percent of women more than 75 years of age have hypertension. In premenopausal women hypertension leads to a tenfold increase in rate of death from CHD.

Diabetes

Women with diabetes are more likely to develop CHD than either men or women without diabetes. For individuals 50 to 59 years of age, diabetes is a greater risk factor for CHD in women than in men. Overall, the relative risk ratio for women with diabetes to develop CHD is 3.5, compared with 2.4 for men with diabetes. Women with diabetes are more likely to die following a MI than women without diabetes or men.

Diabetes eliminates the "protection" that the premenopausal state provides for women. Women usually develop CHD 10 years later than men, but diabetic women lose that decade lag and develop CHD in their 40s. Premenopausal women with diabetes have a sevenfold increase in CHD, which is equal to men in their 40s.

Sedentary Lifestyle

A sedentary lifestyle is a risk factor for CHD in women. The risk decreases in women who exercise.

Oral Contraceptive Pills

The use of estrogen-containing oral contraceptive pills (OCPs) does not increase the risk of CHD. In fact, OCPs may reduce the incidence and risk of CHD (Fig. 5.2). Users of OCPs who did not smoke had one-half the degree of coronary artery plaque as nonusers, as seen on cardiac catheterization in one study. MIs are rare in users of OCPs and only occur in OCP users who are older than age 35 and smoke. The new lower-dose OCPs cause a 15% to 40% increase in triglyceride levels, with a 5% to 10% increase in HDL cholesterol levels. Because HDL has a better predictive value for CHD in women, OCPs may actually lower the risk of CHD in women.

Menopause

The National Cholesterol Education Program (NCEP) recognizes postmenopausal status as a risk factor for CHD, independent of age and weight. Menopause is associated with changes in lipoproteins, including increased LDL and decreased HDL cholesterol levels.

Hormone Replacement Therapy

The Rochester CHD Project, one of the earliest prospective projects that included women, showed that use of estrogen reduced CHD in women 40 to 59 years of age. Estrogen also affect lipids. Hormone replacement therapy (HRT) preserve premenopausal cholesterol profiles and reduce a woman's chances of CHD. HRT also protected against CHD, and the protection was greatest among women with the highest risk for coronary artery disease. There was a 50% reduction in CHD, and a 52% reduction in mortality rates in healthy women without CHD who used HRT. The overall protection effects are attenuated, but typically present at 10 years of HRT use.

However, the Heart and Estrogen/Progestin Replacement Study trial found no decrease in CHD mortality in women who already had CHD for more than 5 years at the time HRT was started. There was an increase in venous thrombotic events of 4.1/1,000 woman-years. Other studies (such as the Nurses Health Study) may have included women who were more likely to do other things to reduce risk (e.g., exercise and/or eating a healthy diet).

Using HRT may also reduce the risk of death caused by CHD-related events. Women who took estrogen had a risk of death of MI in the hospital that was half of that of nonusers of HRT. Women who were using HRT postmenopausally and who were going to have angioplasty had a lower incidence of death or MI, and superior event-free survival.

In many studies, women who use long-term HRT are more likely to demonstrate a "healthy" lifestyle. They are more likely to be of ideal body weight, eat a low-fat and low-calorie diet, and exercise. This makes drawing conclusions difficult.

HRT in more than 30 case control and cohort studies has been shown to decrease risk of CHD, and HRT provides more benefit to women who already have CHD. However, in an individual woman 50 years of age who has no risk factors, the risk of CHD or MI may be smaller than the risks of HRT itself. Decisions about use of HRT must be collaborative and individualized.

Stratification of Risk

Women without any major determinant (no diabetes mellitus, no typical chest pain, and no peripheral vascular disease) have the lowest risk, and fewer than 20% have a likelihood of CHD disease. Women with two or more major, or one major with more than one intermediate or minor, risk factors (Table 5.2 and Fig. 5.2) were at the highest likelihood of CHD (80%).

Prevention

Primary Prevention

Research into primary prevention of CHD in women usually targeted a particular risk factor (Table 5.3). Although obesity is a risk factor for CHD, losing weight does not decrease the risk of developing CHD. Studies have shown that diet and exercise combined can reduce LDL cholesterol in women, but whether these reductions have an effect on CHD morbidity and mortality is not known. Primary prophylactic aspirin therapy may be used in women with risk factors for CHD who are older than 50 years of age, although there have been no prospective trials supporting their use. Although the evidence is still conflicting, use of estrogen may be shown to prevent CHD.

Secondary Prevention

The HERS trial (Heart and Estrogen/Progestin Replacement Study) could not prove that estrogen use was beneficial in reducing further coronary events in women with CHD. Several small trials in postmenopausal women with CHD support the beneficial use of HRT.

T ABLE 5.2. Risk factors of heart disease that are better predictors in women than in men

Risk factor	Better Predictor in Women
Menopause	Yes
Surgical	Yes
Use of oral contraceptive pills	No
Major determinants	
Typical angina pectoris	Yes
Diabetes mellitus	Yes
Peripheral vascular disease	Yes
Intermediate determinants	
Hypertension	Yes, in elderly women
Smoking	No
Lipoproteins	
Low HDL	Yes
Total cholesterol	No
Triglycerides	No
Minor determinants	
Age > 65	No
Obesity	Yes
Sedentary lifestyle	Unknown
Family history	Yes
High stress, low control	Yes

Data from Douglas PS, Ginsburg GS. The evaluation of chest pain in women. *N Engl J Med* 1996;334:1311.

T ABLE 5.3.   Prevention of coronary heart disease in women

Preventive strategies	Supporting evidence
Primary	
Reduce LDL, reduce cholesterol, and increase HDL by diet, exercise, and medication	Fair evidence
Reduction of triglycerides	Some evidence
Aspirin use	No evidence
Use of estrogen/hormone replacement therapy	Fair evidence but conflicting
Secondary	
Use of estrogen/hormone replacement therapy	Disputed evidence
Aspirin	Some evidence

The original trials on the use of aspirin to prevent further coronary events in individuals with CHD either did not include women, did not have a significant number of women, or did not analyze the data by gender. Recent studies suggest that low-dose aspirin benefits men and women with history of occlusive vascular disease by decreasing the risk of subsequent vascular events by 25%. In the setting of an acute MI, aspirin benefits both men and women, reducing the number of fatal and nonfatal events. There was a 32% reduction in the risk of further nonfatal MIs with the use of aspirin.

Other risk factors should be considered as well. Improvement in HDL cholesterol levels and smoking cessation should be strongly addressed. Use of HRT to improve risk in healthy women should be addressed individually, whereas its use in women with CHD for secondary prevention may be more important.

The benefit of aspirin as primary prevention has not been proven in women, but its low side effects and positive secondary prevention suggest it is appropriate for daily use in women older than 50 years of age until long-term studies are available.

Women may present with atypical chest pain or different symptoms from those of men. If a woman has diabetes, she should be evaluated as rigorously as a man. Electrocardiographs and stress testing are important. Treatment modalities including percutaneous transluminal coronary angioplasty (PTCA) and coronary artery bypass grafting (CABG) should be pursued as rigorously as in men.

Further studies are essential, and the behaviors of women and physicians may change when the results are known.

DIAGNOSIS

Differences have been reported in the diagnostic course of women and men who have had similar symptoms. The "usual" modes for diagnosis of CHD in men are the electrocardiogram, echocardiography, the exercise treadmill test (ETT), ETT with thallium or other imaging dyes, and cardiac catheterization (the gold standard). The expense increases with the invasiveness of the test. Cardiac catheterization, although very diagnostically accurate, has problems: it is invasive, requires hospitalization, is expensive, and may cause renal bleeding or vascular complications.

Most studies have examined the question of whether a diagnostic test actually is as accurate, sensitive, and specific in women as in men. Most studies have concluded that there is little difference. As with men, the question is not, "Can this test be used to diagnose CHD?" but, "When should it be used, and in what populations?" The answer is seldom "all women."

Electrocardiographs

Electrocardiographs are as sensitive in women as in men for the diagnosis of heart disease.

Risk Stratification

First, the quality of the chest pain and the number of risk factors can determine the likelihood that a woman has heart disease (Fig. 5.4). The history of the chest pain in a woman with heart disease should be determined. With typical unstable angina, hospitalization is necessary. For women with typical angina by history, the likelihood of CHD is high. For women with atypical chest pain, the likelihood is intermediate, and with nonspecific chest pain, the likelihood is low.

In low-risk women with the least likelihood of having CHD, test results are more likely to be false-positive and should be avoided. However, women with a high likelihood of CHD should undergo routine ETT without nuclear or echocardiograph features unless special situations occur (Fig. 5.4). Many believe that the low specificity of exercise electrocardiography in women precludes its use in women.

Likelihood of Coronary Heart Disease

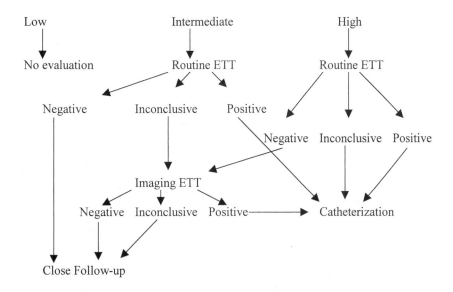

FIGURE 5.4. Evaluation of women with chest pain. ETT, exercise treadmill test. (Data from Douglas PS, Ginsburg GS. The evaluation of chest pain in women. *N Engl J Med* 1996;334:1311.)

Using this algorithm, women are stratified by the likelihood of having CHD, dependent on risk factors, pain, and symptom characteristics. Routine ETT is used only for women with a moderate or high likelihood of having CHD. Imaging ETT is used only for inconclusive ETT in women with moderate risk. All women with positive ETTs should undergo catheterization.

Specialized Exercise Treadmill Testing

Further use of echocardiography during exercise has been proposed for women with a moderate risk of disease. This would increase sensitivity and is less expensive than thallium stress testing. It can also be used if baseline electrocardiographs are abnormal. Images are limited in obese patients. Dobutamine stress echocardiography gave a high sensitivity, specificity, and accuracy in men and women and it was uninfluenced by gender. Dobutamine stress echocardiography was more sensitive in multivessel disease. Technetium Tc99m sestamibi scan testing can be used as well.

REFERRAL

Cardiac Catheterizations

Cardiac catheterization (CC) is the gold standard. Studies 5 to 10 years ago found that men are more likely than women to be referred for CC, perhaps because women have more signs and symptoms that are nonspecific or because they have less serious disease. More recent studies have confirmed that men are still more likely to be referred. The latest study found that physicians estimate the probability of CHD to be lower in women and younger patients. Women and African-American patients were less likely to be referred for CC than white men. In men and women with a similar prevalence of abnormal results on initial stress test, additional studies were performed in only 38% of women compared with 62.3% of men. The indications for CC in women are high index of suspicion of CHD, or intermediate indication for suspicion with a positive ETT, high-risk findings, or persistent pain when ETT is negative or inconclusive (Fig. 5.4).

TREATMENT

Women are less likely to receive thrombolytic agents or to undergo cardiac angiographic intervention or surgical procedures, perhaps because they are older, delay seeking care, or have comorbid conditions, worse disease, or contraindications. Even when eligible, women are still less likely to receive thrombolytic therapy.

Medical Treatment

Chronic medical treatment for angina or CHD in women is similar to that in men, including beta blockers, calcium channel blockers, and nitrates (Table 5.4). In the stable patient who does not have severe disease, there is no difference in mortality in medical or surgical treatment. However, women are less likely to be given emergency medications for acute or unstable angina.

There is no evidence that any particular antianginal medication is more or less effective in women. Women should be treated similarly to men. Recent studies suggested that short-acting calcium channel blockers used in men and women for hypertension increased the risk of mortality from cardiovascular disease.

Women are less likely to receive intravenous nitroglycerin, heparin, or thrombolysis.

Surgical Treatment

Women are less likely to have interventional PTCA than men with similar symptoms. One study looked at which women had angioplasty. Women, as a group, had a higher prevalence of unstable angina, congestive heart failure (CHF), diabetes, hypertension, and noncardiac illnesses at the time of angioplasty than men who had angioplasty. These women were at higher surgical risk and had higher rates of inoperable disease than men. Men were more likely to have abnormal left ventricular function and a his-

T ABLE 5.4. Medical therapy for angina

Agent	Method of Delivery	Comments
Nitrates	PO, pill SL, spray SL, daily patches	Use-free intervals are necessary; 10% do not respond; 10% have severe headaches
Beta blockers	PO	20% do not respond; cannot be used in individuals with asthma, respiratory problems, diabetes, depression, bronchospasm
CCBs	PO	Short-acting CCB may be associated with increased risk of MI; can cause heart blocks, CHF
Aspirin	PO 80–300 mg daily	Primary and secondary prevention, but only proven effective in men

Abbreviations: CCB, calcium channel blockers; CHF, congestive heart failure; MI, myocardial infarction; SL, sublingual.

tory of MI, and CABG surgery. Even so, the outcomes were similar; approximately 40% of women and men had complete revascularization, but women were more likely to have complications.

It is unclear why a difference in referral rates exists. Women have more complicated CHD when they receive PTCA and/or are poor candidates for bypass surgery. There may be a bias toward taking a woman's disease less seriously or treating women longer with medication before suggesting PTCA. When women receive PTCA, they do as well as men, or better.

Women with coronary artery disease are less likely to undergo CABG and are likely to be referred for it later. Women are likely to be older and sicker at time of surgery, just as with PTCA. At the time of referral for CABG, they are more likely to have angina, CHF, hypertension, and diabetes. In the Systolic Hypertension in the Elderly Program (SHEP), older patients and women, regardless of comorbid conditions, underwent less intensive cardiovascular intervention than younger patients and men.

There are no data on how decisions are made for when to refer a woman for CABG. Not one of the major trials provided clear data from which specific indications for CABG in women can be determined.

Mortality rates for women after CABG have been reported to be higher, with as much as four times greater in-hospital mortality than that in men. In several studies women have a higher operative mortality rate (1.3% to 8.8%) than men (0.9% to 3%). The fact that women are referred later in the course of disease may account for the higher in-hospital mortality in women following CABG, regardless of age, urgency of surgery, and state of left ventricular systolic function. Women have more risk factors when they are referred for CABG, such as advanced age, unstable angina, previous MI, diabetes, advanced functional class, and small-caliber coronary arteries. Women were more likely than men to be single and live alone. Women have smaller arteries, which may lead to excessive technical difficulties. Several studies suggest that when adjusted for vessel size, variance, and baseline clinical and angiographic profiles, female gender alone did not remain a statistically significant risk factor. Smaller vessel size, rather than gender, seems to explain the higher mortality rate.

Women are more likely to have diabetes and CHD. Diabetes is a good predictor of increased mortality after bypass surgery because the autonomic dysfunction and neuropathy can cause silent MIs and higher risks of cardiac arrhythmias and respiratory failures.

CABG in women is less effective. Data suggest that grafts in women reocclude faster, and women are less likely to derive anginal relief from CABG.

Women are less likely to be referred for cardiac rehabilitation after CABG.

SUGGESTED READING

Stefanick ML, Mackey S, Sheehan M, et al. Effects of diet and exercise in men and post-menopausal women with low levels of HDL cholesterol and high levels of LDL cholesterol. *N Engl J Med* 1998:339;12.

CHAPTER 6

Weight-Related Issues

C. Carolyn Thiedke

OBESITY

Regardless of the reason a woman visits her physician, she frequently has concerns about her weight. She may desperately want help with this problem yet be reluctant to mention it out of embarrassment or fear of disapproval.

Two factors are important. First, the prevalence of obesity is increasing in all age groups and both genders in most developed nations. Second, our society holds up to women what is for most an unobtainable ideal body image, which is thinner than what is medically ideal. This disparity between the real and the ideal is a source of great psychic stress for many women of all ages, income levels, and professions.

In the United States there are three commonly held beliefs among physicians and the public:
- Being overweight is always bad for one's health.
- Obesity is always due to uncontrolled eating.
- Anyone who wants to be thin can be.

These beliefs contribute to the stigmatization of those who are obese and give support to the multimillion-dollar weight loss industry.

In one study of patients who had lost 100 pounds (45 kg) or more after gastric bypass, many patients indicated they would rather be an amputee or be blind, deaf, or dyslexic than to return to their former weights. All participants stated that they would decline a multimillionaire lifestyle if it meant returning to their obese status.

Chief Complaint
- A 35-year-old woman presents for a physical examination and lists a desire to lose weight among her concerns. She exercises several times a week and tries to eat less but is frustrated by no change on the scale. She is otherwise healthy.

Clinical Manifestations
The signs of obesity are obvious and the symptoms are well known:
- Clothing that constricts
- Limbs and a midsection that undulate with walking or running
- Breathlessness and muscle fatigue at levels of exertion once done easily
- Chafing and irritation of parts of the body that rub together
- Shame felt when meeting new people or entering new situations
- Ruminations of guilt and frustration over one's inability to cut back on caloric intake or to exercise regularly
- Arthritic symptoms, particularly in the larger joints, like hips and knees
- Sleep-related symptoms such as snoring or apneic episodes

Other conditions that are related to obesity include venous stasis disease, gastroesophageal reflux disease, and stress urinary incontinence.

The physical examination of an obese patient should include height and weight for the purpose of calculating body mass index (BMI). The pattern of fat distribution,

85

whether predominantly central body (or "apple-shaped") or predominantly lower body (or "pear-shaped"), has become a critical distinction in assessing the risks associated with obesity. The simple maneuver of measuring the waistline gives a reasonable estimate of this distinction. In women a waistline of more than 35 inches (88 cm) is correlated with this more adverse central obesity.

In addition to the obvious corpulence, findings may include the following:
• Intertrigo
• Joint deformities related to osteoarthritis
• Polycystic ovarian syndrome with its stigmata is the most common endocrine disorder of reproduction that is associated with obesity

Other physical findings related to the cardiovascular and metabolic consequences of obesity will be covered in the section entitled "Metabolic Syndrome."

Epidemiology

Obesity, as defined by a BMI of more than 30 kg/m^2, is commonly found in all developed nations. The prevalence of obesity in both adults and children is increasing at a rate considered alarming by medical and public health experts. The most recent analysis from the third National Health and Nutrition Examination Survey (NHANES III) indicated that 35% of all American adults (20 years of age or older) are overweight. In addition, 14% of children between the ages of 6 and 11, and 12% of adolescents between the ages of 12 and 17 are overweight.

In the United States more than 30% of adults are considered obese. The rate is higher in some ethnic populations such as African- and Mexican-Americans and alarmingly high among those from the Pacific Islands—approaching 65% to 80%. Rates are somewhat lower in most European countries, and in New Zealand, Canada, and Australia.

Risk Factors

Considerable attention has been paid over the past several years to calculating the role that genetics plays in obesity. Although it is clear that obesity tends to run in families, no consensus exists regarding which factor plays the greater role—genetics or family environment.

Studies comparing obesity in monozygotic and dizygotic twins suggest that 70% of the variation in body weight is due to genetic inheritance. However, only 20% of those who are obese are considered genetically obese. It is unlikely that we will find a single "obesity gene" for humans. Even when genetic inheritance is a factor, whether or not that gene is expressed depends on other factors, such as environment, stage of development, and gender. Although it is widely assumed that the mechanism by which genes exert their influence is over the metabolic rate, it is just as likely that genes may influence such behaviors as eating and exercise. There has been a widespread assumption that certain psychologic factors put individuals at risk for obesity. These assumptions have arisen because early psychologic studies in obese patients were conducted in patients presenting to treatment programs for obesity. When examining populations at large, there is little evidence that the obese differ from the nonobese in their personality traits. Among those who seek treatment, obese patients generally have poor self-esteem, but this appears to be secondary to the way the obese are perceived by society, and not the cause of the obesity. Among those who seek treatment, a higher percentage of individuals carry an Axis I and II diagnosis. Among the obese, more report a history of rape, sexual molestation, or posttraumatic stress disorder than the general population.

Although being overweight in early childhood does not correlate well with obesity as an adult, by school age, childhood obesity becomes a risk factor for adult obesity. One-half of obese schoolchildren will become obese adults. Thirty percent of obese women were obese as adolescents. Conversely, 70% of obese women were not obese as adolescents.

The current milieu in our society that provides a wide variety of high-fat foods while promoting sedentary behavior accounts for the increasing prevalence of obesity. It is easy to follow the rise in obesity as developing countries become more prosperous and adopt Western lifestyles.

Pathology

Adipose tissue is composed of a number of cell types, including adipocytes, the main fat-containing cells, very small fat cells, fibroblasts, endothelial cells, and blood cells. Considerable research has looked at the rate of proliferation of adipocytes throughout the lifespan.

There appear to be two periods of adipocyte proliferation: one in the first year of life and a smaller one in the years before puberty. Adipose tissue mass is believed to remain relatively stable in adults. Thus expansion of adipose tissue is due to the enlargement of existing cells rather than to the addition of new cells.

It has been thought that weight loss does not alter the number of adipocytes; hence the dismaying tendency for weight to be regained after loss. Two studies in the 1980s, however, have demonstrated a reduction in the number of adipocytes following significant weight loss.

Diagnosis

Although it is easy to determine that someone is overweight by sight, the challenge has been to define obesity and to determine when it is no longer merely an aesthetic problem but a medical concern. The BMI has become the accepted measurement of obesity because it estimates body fat better than the simple measurement of weight. In addition, measuring a patient's waistline with a tape measure estimates central versus peripheral fat deposition, an important determination for assessing health risks. In women, a waistline measurement of more than 35 inches (88 cm) is indicative of central obesity. Numerous other measurements of weight are used in research studies, including skin thickness, absorptiometry, computed tomography, and immersion to calculate percentage body fat, but these are expensive and not widely available.

The World Health Organization (WHO) has made the following determination about BMI and obesity:

- BMI 25.00 to 29.99 kg/mm^2—Overweight
- BMI 30.00 to 34.99 kg/mm^2—Class I obesity
- BMI 35.00 to 39.99 kg/mm^2—Class II obesity
- BMI more than 40.00 kg/mm^2—Class III obesity
  See Table 6.1 and Fig. 6.1.

The presence of comorbid diseases increases the health risk of obesity. Therefore risk factors such as high blood pressure, lipid levels, cigarette smoking, sedentary lifestyle, diabetes, and family history of cardiac disease must be assessed.

Although obesity alone is an infrequent presentation for thyroid disease, screening for thyroid disease may be appropriate, if other symptoms are present.

Referral

An interested family physician can counsel and provide weight loss advice to those who are mildly to moderately overweight. However, most obese individuals in the moderately to severely overweight category need a more intensive program than most physicians have the time or resources to provide. Family physicians should keep apprised of the programs, both commercial and noncommercial, in their area that can provide such care (Table 6.2).

T ABLE 6.1.   Appropriate treatment options for each level of health risk

Level of Health Risk	Appropriate Treatment Option
Minimal or low	Moderate caloric restriction (1,200 kcal/day)
	Increased physical activity
	Behavioral change
Moderate	Above options, plus greater caloric restriction (800–1200 kcal/day)
High and very high	Above options, plus medications and VLCD (<800 kcal/day)
Extremely high	Above options, plus surgical intervention

Abbreviation: VLCD, very-low-calorie diet.

Source: Shape UP America, 6707 Democracy Boulevard, Suite 306, Bethesda, MD 20817; www.shapeup.org.

Management

Weight loss occurs when an energy deficit is created (i.e., when more energy is expended than consumed). A deficit can be created by decreasing caloric intake or by increasing energy expenditure. The most successful programs combine the two. Studies have consistently shown that loss of as little as 5% to 10% of body weight pays dividends in improved blood pressure, improved lipid profiles, and improved insulin resistance. Improved mood and quality of life have been consistent findings in those

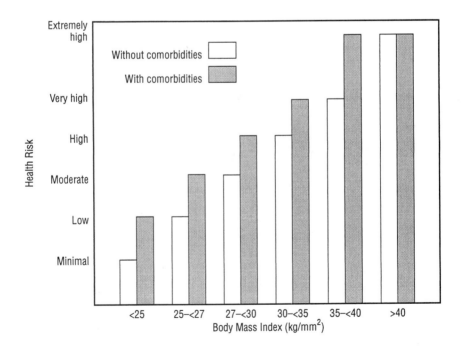

FIGURE 6.1. Association of body mass index and health risks with and without comorbid conditions.

T ABLE 6.2. Weight loss programs

Program	Type	Description	Cost	Contact
TOPS (Take Off Pounds Sensibly) Club, Inc.	Noncommercial	Group support, no specific diet, or exercise	Dues	800-932-8677
OA (Overeaters Anonymous)	Noncommercial	Group support, based on 12-step program	None	Check in local phone book
Diet Workshop	Commercial	Diet, exercise, behavior modification	$169/3 months	800-488-3438
Jenny Craig, Inc.	Commercial	Diet, exercise, behavior modification, requires purchase of foods	Enrollment + $70/week	800-29-JENNY
Weight Watchers International, Inc.	Commercial	Nutrition, exercise, and lifestyle modification	One-time registration fee + weekly meetings	800-651-6000
Health Management Resources (HMR)	Clinical	Low-calorie diet or VLCD with intensive lifestyle education	$150/week	800-418-1367
Medifast	Clinical	Low-calorie diet or VLCD	$65–85/week	800-638-7867
New Direction	Clinical	Moderate-low-calorie diet	$100/week	800-222-9201
Optifast	Clinical	800–950 kcal/day diet	$75–120 week	800-662-2540

Abbreviation: VLCD, very-low-calorie diet.
Source: Shape Up America!

who have lost a significant amount of weight. Patients embarking on a weight loss program should be encouraged to set reasonable, attainable goals that improve health rather than to focus on goals based on an aesthetic ideal that is often more difficult to attain. It cannot be stressed enough that successful maintenance of weight loss is possible only in the context of lifelong behavior changes.

Weight loss strategies can be thought of as a tripod. A change in dietary habits is often considered the first step in any weight loss program. Diets can be classified by the degree of caloric restriction:
• 1,200 kcal/day (for women)—Moderate-deficit diet
• 800 to 1,200 kcal/day (for women)—Low-calorie diet
• Less than 800 kcal/day (for women)—Very-low-calorie diet

The very-low-calorie diet is not advisable outside of a closely supervised medical setting. Patients can attempt the other two on their own or through a commercial or noncommercial weight loss program.

Some commercial programs provide structured meals. A few studies have shown higher initial weight loss with structured meals but no difference in long-term maintenance. Any caloric restriction should be well balanced with adequate amounts of protein and carbohydrates. Using the U.S. Department of Agriculture Food Pyramid as a model provides patients with a structure to guide their eating habits.

Counting calories may seem too complicated to many patients. Physicians should have alternate suggestions for patients who seem easily discouraged. Other strategies have been shown to be effective in promoting weight loss. Some have suggested that lowering the percentage of fat in the diet, rather than overall caloric restriction, represents an appropriate dietary strategy. Indeed, one study comparing fat restriction with caloric restriction found that although weight loss was not different, women on the low-fat diet showed better adherence to dietary guidelines and rated the diet as more palatable. Another recent study found weight loss with restricting only certain types of calorically dense, nutritionally poor foods (beef, hot dogs, concentrated sweets). One approach, probably most successful with those who are only mildly to moderately overweight, is to make people more aware of portion sizes (Tables 6.3 and 6.4). Patients can be asked to visualize their plate as divided into quarters. Their serving of meat should take up only one-quarter of the plate; their starch, only one-quarter; and their vegetables, one-half.

The second leg of the weight loss tripod is exercise. Exercise alone has not been associated with significant weight loss; however, it is key to long-term maintenance of weight loss. Patients who exercise show better maintenance of weight loss at 1 year than do those who do not exercise. Physical activity is associated with decreases in all-cause mortality at any BMI. The most impressive effect is in those whose BMI is more than 30 kg/mm^2. Recent research has shown the benefit of a lifestyle approach to exercise rather than the traditionally recommended structured activity program. Subjects were encouraged to find ways throughout their daily routine to become more active (e.g., taking the stairs; parking farther away from their destination; taking breaks during the day to take short, brisk walks; engaging more often in strenuous household chores such as vacuuming, washing the car, and gardening). After 6 months, people in the lifestyle arm of the study showed health benefits equal to those in the structured activity program.

Recent recommendations from the Centers for Disease Control and Prevention and the American College of Sports Medicine call for 30 minutes of accumulated activity most days of the week. In one study, women were instructed to take four 10-minute exercise breaks per day; another group was instructed to perform all its exercise in one 40-minute time period. At the end of the study, the former group had significantly more minutes of exercise more days of the week and had lost more weight.

The third leg of the weight loss tripod is behavior change. To be successful in weight loss, patients must be willing to look at the behaviors that promote their obesity and adopt new ones that will help them lose weight.

The following are essential components of a behavioral strategy:

- Self-monitoring. Although often perceived as onerous by patients, keeping track of caloric intake and exercise enhances the chance that weight loss will be maintained.

T ABLE 6.3.   USDA food pyramid serving sizes

Food Groups	Serving Size	Visual Representation
Meat, poultry, fish	2–3 oz., cooked	Deck of cards, palm of hand
Vegetables	1 cup	Size of fist
Fruit	1 medium	Size of baseball
Rice or pasta	$^1/_2$ cup, cooked	Scoop of ice cream
Cheese	1 $^1/_2$ oz	Pair of dice or dominoes
Oil	use sparingly	Tip of thumb
Dry cereal	1 oz.	Large handful

TABLE 6.4. Recommended servings of each food group for various caloric intakes

	Number of Portions		
Food Group	1,200 kcal/day	1,600 kcal/day	2,000 kcal/day
Dairy (milk, yogurt, cheese, soy)	2	3	3
Protein (meat, fish, poultry, beans)	4	5	6
Grain (bread, rice, pasta, cereal)	5	6	8
Vegetable	3	4	5
Fruit	2	3	4
Extras: Fats, oils, sweets	4	6	8

- Realistic goal setting.
- Adoption of healthier eating habits.
- Establishment of a regular exercise routine.
- Stimulus control.

As soon as goal behaviors have been identified, patients must determine what they need to do to achieve those behaviors. The environment should be altered to make healthy behaviors more likely; for instance, having exercise attire immediately at hand and making negative behaviors less likely, such as ridding the house of high-calorie snack food. The following are also helpful:

- **Problem solving.** Patients are encouraged to anticipate situations that lead to overeating (e.g., parties, stress, or underexercising) and to plan how they will cope with them.
- **Cognitive restructuring.** Patients learn to resist the negative thoughts, such as hopelessness, shame, rationalizations, and comparing themselves with others, that sabotage diet attempts.
- **Relapse prevention.** Patients are taught to distinguish lapses from relapses as a means of avoiding feelings of failure and dropping out.

Behavioral programs that emphasize these behaviors can lead to weight losses of 18 to 20 pounds (8 to 9 kg) over a few months.

Medication may be appropriate for those who are moderately to severely obese (Table 6.5). To decide if drug treatment is appropriate, calculation of the BMI is necessary, as is an assessment of fat distribution, estimated by measuring the waist. Having a waist circumference between 28 and 35 inches (71 to 90 cm) moves up the patient's health risk a category (e.g., from low to moderate or moderate to high) and having a waist size greater than 35 inches (88 cm) moves up the patient's risk two categories. Drugs affect weight by one of three mechanisms:

- Decreasing food intake
- Boosting metabolism
- Increasing energy expenditure

Surgical treatment of obesity remains a realistic option for patients whose BMI exceeds 40 kg/mm^2 or those with a BMI of more than 35 kg/mm^2 and serious comorbidity (Table 6.6). Kral, writing in the *Handbook of Obesity*, states, "The risks of the currently perfected techniques are so low and the benefits, whether in terms of morbidity reduction, quality of life improvement, patient satisfaction, or mortality reduction, are so convincing that surgical treatment of obesity must be considered an established and legitimate form of treatment."

T ABLE 6.5.   Selected agents for the treatment of obesity

Agent (Trade Name)	Mechanism	Daily Dose (mg)
Diethylpropion	Centrally active adrenergic	
Tenuate		75
Tenuate dospan		75
Mazindol	Centrally active adrenergic	
Sanorex		1–3
Mazanor		1–3
Phentermine HCL	Centrally active adrenergic	
Adipex-P		37.5
Fastin		30
Obe-Nix		37.5
Zantryl		30
Phentermine resin Ionamin		30
Sibutramine Meridia	Combined adrenergic and serotonergic	10–15
Orlistat Xenical	Inhibits absorption of fat	360

In the most complete study available, 83% of patients with type 2 diabetes treated with surgical intervention were maintaining normal blood glucose and glycosolated hemoglobins at an average follow-up of 7.6 years. In that same study, the rate of hypertension dropped to 14% postoperatively, from a rate of 58% preoperatively among those who had had surgery. Other improvements noted after surgery include the following:
• Improvements in ventricular functioning
• Reduction in myocardial thickness and chamber size
• Sustained normalization of lipid profiles
• Reduction in sleep apneic episodes
• Improved quality of life
• Patients formerly receiving disability or public assistance returned to work

T ABLE 6.6.   Surgical interventions in the treatment of obesity

	Body Weight Lost (%)	Perioperative Risk (%)	Complications
Vertical plastic binding (VBG)	40–63	0–1.0	Leak, sepsis, outlet stenosis, peptic ulceration, staple disruption, revision rate 41% to 45%
Roux-en-y gastric bypass (RYGB)	68–72	0.5–1.0	Outlet stenosis, leak, sepsis, anemia, vitamin or mineral deficiencies

Source: Kral JG. Surgical treatment of obesity. In: Bray GA, ed. *Handbook of Obesity.* New York: Marcel Dekker, 1998.

Several conditions would temporarily exclude someone from considering weight loss:
- Pregnancy
- Lactation
- Unstable mental illness
- Unstable medical illness
  Other conditions that require clinical judgment include the following:
- Osteoporosis. Caloric restriction appears to hasten bone loss either through decreased intake of calcium or through loss of muscle mass.
- Cholelithiasis. Weight loss appears to predispose to symptomatic gallstones.
  A few conditions are absolute contraindications to weight loss:
- Anorexia nervosa
- Terminal illness
- HIV/AIDS

Follow-up

Physicians who decide to treat an obese individual instead of referring her to a weight loss program must understand that regular follow-up is essential. Every 2 to 4 weeks is appropriate at the outset, with longer intervals as weight loss stabilizes. For physicians who prescribe medication as part of a weight loss program or in conjunction with a commercial or noncommercial weight loss program, follow-up is needed monthly to monitor progress and to watch for the appearance of side effects.

Patients who decline assistance for weight loss should be instructed in ways of avoiding further weight gain, such as increasing their activity or making dietary changes. At subsequent visits, these patients should be asked if their feelings about trying to lose weight have changed. Patients who have had a temporary exclusion from weight loss should be evaluated at subsequent visits for a change in that situation.

Although the benefits of weight loss are great, there are some risks for complications:
- Overzealous caloric restriction without proper supplementation of nutrients that can lead to nutritional deficits
- Depression
- Possible further bone loss in women with osteoporosis
- Increased risk of cholelithiasis, although obesity itself is an independent risk factor for gallstones

Patient Education

Physicians must examine their own beliefs about obesity and determine if they retain beliefs that stigmatize the obese. These attitudes can be telegraphed to patients and make a successful partnership for weight loss unlikely. To assess a patient's readiness to consider weight loss, a physician may use the stages of change model devised by Prochaska and his colleagues:
- **Precontemplation.** Patients at this stage are not considering any behavior change. They are either in denial about the health risks of their obesity or so discouraged from previous attempts to lose weight that they are unwilling to try again.
- **Contemplation.** Patients at this stage are aware of their need to lose weight and anticipate an attempt within the next 6 months but are not ready to commit to a change now.

- **Preparation.** Patients at this stage are gathering the information they need to make a change in their behavior.
- **Action.** Patients have launched into their weight loss program.
- **Maintenance.** Patients have reached their goal and are continuing to use the behaviors that allowed them to lose weight.

Physicians can raise the issue of treatment for obesity in a nonjudgmental way that conveys caring and emphasizes the health risks of continued obesity. By doing this skillfully, physicians can help move patients from the stage of precontemplation to contemplation or from contemplation to preparation and action.

Physicians should avoid automatically recommending weight loss to every person who needs to lose a few pounds. Those recommendations should be reserved for those who are severely overweight or who are moderately overweight and have obesity-related disease or other risk factors.

Physicians should convey a sense of optimism about weight loss, emphasizing that modest weight loss, as little as 5% to 10% of initial body weight, can reduce health risks. They should also have at their fingertips resources that expand the counseling they are able to do in their office, such as the following:

- Sample food and exercise diaries
- Behavioral contracts to help patients state explicitly what behaviors they intend to change and how they intend to reward themselves
- Worksheets that help patients determine what situations lead to overeating and how they can circumvent lapses
- Worksheets that assess what exercise program is most suited to that patient's temperament and situation and has the most likely chance of sustained compliance (Table 6.7)
- Handouts that provide dietary recommendations, particularly regarding use of the Food Pyramid, reading food labels, and lowering fat intake
- A list of community resources for weight loss

These resources can be developed by the physician, or adapted from many of the professional organizations that have developed weight loss materials.

Several family physicians, motivated to provide continuity of care around this health issue, offer group classes to their patients to deal with most of the topics listed earlier.

T ABLE 6.7. Questions to ask patients to help them decide which exercise program might work best for them

1. Am I most likely to exercise in the morning or late afternoon/early evening?
2. Am I most comfortable by myself or would finding a "buddy" keep me motivated?
3. Would I rather try this by myself or enroll in a class?
4. Am I on a tight budget, or is buying exercise equipment or joining a gym an option for me?
5. Is hiring a trainer something I would find helpful and affordable?
6. Do I feel safe in my neighborhood or do I need to find another place to exercise?
7. Do I have joint, muscle, or other physical problems that influence my choice of exercise?
8. Do I enjoy being outdoors or would I prefer exercising indoors?
9. Is there some form of exercise I really enjoyed in the past?

BULIMIA AND BINGE-EATING DISORDER

Bulimia nervosa and binge-eating disorder (BED) are the two most common eating disorders. The third is anorexia nervosa, which is relatively uncommon. These are psychophysiologic disturbances stemming from cognitive, affective, and behavioral distortions around food and eating behavior.

In bulimia nervosa, a woman engages in frequent bouts of binge eating that lead to significant emotional distress. This leads to compensatory behaviors to avoid weight gain. Self-induced vomiting is the most common behavior (80% to 90%), followed by laxative use (35% to 75%). Other behaviors include overuse of diuretics, thyroid hormone, anorexiant medications, and enemas, or the use of ipecac.

BED is also associated with frequent episodes of eating large amounts over a short period of time. It too is accompanied by emotional distress, often a feeling of loss of control, but the compensatory behaviors listed earlier are absent.

Chief Complaints

- A 19-year-old college student on an athletic scholarship in diving tearfully admits that she purges on a regular basis to maintain her weight at the level stipulated by her coach.
- A 37-year-old severely obese secretary acknowledges that she often consumes large amounts of food furtively when her family is not around.

Clinical Manifestations

Depending on the severity of the eating disorder, there may be little or no physical findings. Women who are bulimic may be below, at, or above ideal weight.

Women with BED are more often overweight. They are more likely than obese, nonbinging women to present complaining of gastrointestinal complaints such as bloating, abdominal pain, nausea, and vomiting. For women who engage regularly in purging, there may be subtle signs on physical examination:
- Parotid enlargement
- Erosion of the lingual surface of the teeth and multiple caries from frequent exposure of the teeth to stomach acid
- Scarring may be noted on the dorsum of the hand from repeated attempts to induce vomiting
- A Mallory-Weiss tear of the esophagus (infrequent)

Epidemiology

The prevalence of bulimia has been estimated at 1% to 3% of women of high school and college age, although the number of people who engage in these behaviors less frequently and thus do not meet diagnostic criteria is probably much greater. Bulimia is found among all ethnic, racial, and sociocultural groups. BED probably affects 2% to 3% of the general population but becomes more common with increasing weight. It is thought to affect 5% of the obese in community populations, 10% to 15% of the mildly obese in commercial weight loss programs, and up to 50% of morbidly obese patients seeking bariatric surgery. Studies have shown an earlier onset for BED than for bulimia (14.3 versus 19.8 years).

Risk Factors

Patients with eating disorders have high rates of depression and high rates of a family history of depression. It is not completely clear, however, whether the depression is primary or secondary. Obsessive-compulsive disorder is more prevalent in patients with bulimia than in the general population, as are rates of related disorders, generalized anxiety disorder, and phobias. Personality disorders involving impulsivity are found more frequently in those with eating disorders than in control subjects. Substance abuse disorders are more frequent among binge eaters. A biologic predisposition to eating disorders is postulated based either on neuroendocrine or physiologic abnormalities but has not been proved. Sexual abuse has been postulated as a precipitant of eating disorders, but the rate does not appear to be any higher than that in the population with psychiatric disorders in general. Although there is no evidence that binge eaters are "addicted" to certain foods, such as sugars or carbohydrates, one research study showed that binge eaters selectively decreased their intake of these foods when given naloxone.

Diagnosis

Table 6.8 lists the DSM-IV criteria for bulimia nervosa and BED. Lab test abnormalities may include hypokalemia, hyperamylasemia, and metabolic alkalosis.

Referral

For patients whose episodes of binging and purging are relatively infrequent and not of long duration, a family physician motivated to provide care may be of great service in helping delineate the scope of the problem and providing treatment. However, most patients who meet DSM-IV criteria may require the services of a specialist in eating disorders who can provide psychotherapy and medication. Overeaters Anonymous and other support groups can be of immense help to these patients.

Management

Bulimia can generally be managed in an outpatient setting. Both psychotherapy and medication have been found to be useful. Cognitive behavioral therapy (CBT) is the best-studied treatment and is generally considered the treatment of choice. Individuals are taught to examine the beliefs and feelings that lead to binging and purging, and to consciously alter them. Review articles have shown a decrease in the frequency of episodes by 79% to 86% at the end of treatment, and about half of patients have stopped binging and purging altogether. Fluoxetine (Prozac) at a dosage of 60

T ABLE 6.8.   DSM-IV criteria for eating disorders

I. Bulimia nervosa
   A. Recurrent episodes of binge eating
   B. Recurrent inappropriate compensatory behaviors to prevent weight gain
   C. The binge eating and inappropriate compensatory behaviors both occur, on average, at least twice weekly for 3 months
   D. Self-evaluation is unduly influenced by body weight and shape
   E. Type: Purging, nonpurging
II. Binge-eating disorder
   A. Recurrent episodes of binge eating
   B. The binge eating episodes are associated with at least three behavioral indicators of loss of control
   C. Marked distress regarding binge eating
   D. The binge eating occurs, on average, at least twice weekly for 6 months
   E. The binge eating is not associated with the regular use of inappropriate compensatory behaviors and does not occur exclusively during the course of anorexia nervosa or bulimia nervosa

mg/day was shown to be more effective than placebo, though many patients were still binging at the end of the 8-week treatment and relapse rates were as high as 50% at 4 weeks, despite continuous drug treatment. For BED, both interpersonal and CBT have been found to reduce binging episodes. Because many with BED are also overweight, enrollment in a standard weight loss program is often desirable. Antidepressants have been tried in BED, but proof of efficacy is lacking. Treatment programs for BED emphasize behavioral changes such as the following:
• Avoid the purchase of binge foods while grocery shopping
• Plan ahead for alternate behavior under stressful situations
• Delay consumption when the urge to binge strikes by engaging in alternate behaviors
    Additional instructions for binging patients include the following:
• Avoid deprivation
• Eat regularly spaced meals and snacks
• Have a small amount of fat at every meal to promote satiety

Follow-up

Both bulimia and BED should be considered chronic, relapsing diseases in which symptoms may improve but seldom disappear. Family physicians caring for women with eating disorders should establish a sense of trust with the patient and inquire about relapses on a regular basis. In patients with bulimia, physicians should be vigilant for serious medical complications, such as electrolyte disturbances and cardiomyopathy secondary to ipecac abuse.

Patient Education

Patients should be told that although these eating disorders are generally lifelong conditions, treatment is available to help them regain a sense of control over their eating and, hence, their lives. Physicians should forge a trusting relationship with these patients so that they will feel free to ask for help when they relapse.

METABOLIC SYNDROME

Previously known as Syndrome X, plurimetabolic syndrome, and the "deadly quartet" (insulin resistance, dyslipidemia, hypertension, and central obesity), this is a cluster of several metabolic abnormalities that taken together increase a person's risk for cardiovascular disease, diabetes, and stroke. Metabolic syndrome is included in this chapter because of the recognition that a pattern of central or abdominal obesity is a key feature of the syndrome. Insulin resistance is considered by most to be the sine qua non of the metabolic syndrome.

Chief Complaint

• A 57-year-old divorced parking lot attendant presents for routine follow-up of her diabetes and hypertension. Her glycosolated hemoglobin level and blood pressure level reveal poor control. She is dismayed because of a steady weight gain over the past year that has resulted in her clothes fitting poorly. You calculate her BMI at 32 kg/m^2.

Clinical Manifestations

The signs and symptoms of metabolic syndrome are the same as those for obesity (listed earlier in the chapter). In women, a waist measurement of greater than 35 inches (88 cm) indicates central obesity. In addition, these patients have elevated blood sugar levels, elevated blood pressures levels, and dyslipidemia (elevated very-

low-density lipoprotein [VLDL] combined with low high-density lipoprotein [HDL]). Other factors that are frequently associated with metabolic syndrome but not a part of the definition include the following:
- Hyperuricemia
- Sedentary lifestyle
- Hyperandrogenism
- Growth hormone deficiency
- Tobacco use

Epidemiology

The prevalence of metabolic syndrome has been difficult to establish because of the lack of a standardized definition. Using insulin resistance as a single criterion, it is probable that 25% of populations that follow a typical Western lifestyle of overconsumption of high-fat, high-carbohydrate foods are affected. Studies that have looked at central obesity as defined by waist-to-hip ratio (WHR) as a marker for metabolic syndrome estimate that about 20% of such populations are affected.

Risk Factors

Certain ethnic groups, such as the Pima Indians, aboriginal Australians, and some Pacific Islanders, have remarkably high rates of metabolic syndrome. Metabolic syndrome becomes more prevalent with advancing age. Central pattern obesity is more common in men than in women, who more commonly display gynoid or peripheral obesity. In women, however, with central obesity, it may be even more devastating than in men. Genetic predisposition to hypertension has been recognized for some time. Recent studies have identified a genetic locus that appears to be related to the development of insulin resistance.

Pathology

It appears that metabolic syndrome involves an interplay between multiple factors, including genetics, environment, behavioral factors and neuroendocrine abnormalities that interact to create the deposition of adipose tissue around visceral organs. Although these factors may also act independently, this visceral adiposity leads to the following:
- Decreased insulin sensitivity
- Increased insulin secretion
- Impaired insulin clearance
  These in turn lead to the following:
- Hyperinsulinemia
- Increased triglyceride levels
- Lowered levels of HDL cholesterol
- Greater percentage of LDL cholesterol—the small, dense fraction known as pattern B, which is thought to be more atherogenic
- Hyperglycemia

Diagnosis

Visceral fat appears to be the factor most closely associated with metabolic syndrome. Although abdominal computed tomography (CT) is used in research settings to assess visceral fat, in primary care practice this is not feasible. The WHR has been found to be an accessible, low-cost, accurate substitute measurement for central obesity. A WHR greater than 0.8 indicates central obesity in women, as does waist size greater than 35 inches (88 cm). Elevated systolic and diastolic blood pressure readings are essential for the diagnosis of metabolic syndrome. Other parameters of metabolic syndrome are obtained from biochemical profiles such as a fasting lipid panel showing high triglycerides, high total cholesterol, low HDL cholesterol, high LDL cholesterol, and high VLDL levels. Other findings, not assessed routinely, are high levels of lipoprotein (a) and an LDL pattern B (small, dense particles). As obesity worsens, so does hyperinsulinemia, leading to overt type 2 diabetes with elevated fasting blood glucose and glycosylated hemoglobin levels.

Referral

Family physicians are well able to manage the sequelae of metabolic syndrome, including treatment of hypertension, normalization of blood glucose, and treatment of hyperlipidemia. As mentioned in the section on obesity, physicians may want to work with a dietitian in helping patients lose weight. Physicians may want to refer those with very high triglycerides, poorly controlled diabetes, or evidence of worsening macrovascular disease.

Management

Weight loss is tantamount to successful treatment of metabolic syndrome. In a study of obese individuals, after an average weight loss of 19.8 pounds (9 kg), 50% of those with glucose intolerance had normalized their blood glucose levels. Decreased caloric intake with subsequent weight loss markedly improves insulin resistance and the other metabolic markers of this syndrome. The American Diabetes Association says, "There is no one 'diabetic diet.'" To promote compliance with dietary recommendations, food plans should be individualized as much as possible to consider ethnic, regional, and personal preferences.

Recent studies have looked at the glycemic index of foods. The glycemic index is a useful tool that measures how fast a food is likely to raise blood glucose. Foods with high glycemic index (e.g., highly processed foods such as white bread, sugary cereals, pasta, bagels) raise blood glucose levels quickly and appear to be associated with excess food intake (Table 6.9). A diet of foods with low glycemic index (e.g., legumes,

T ABLE 6.9. Glycemic index of selected foods

High glycemic index
  White bread
  Corn flakes
  Bagels
Moderately high glycemic index
  Banana
  Brown rice
  Carrots
Moderately low glycemic index
  Apples
  Peas
  Pinto beans
Low glycemic index
  Broccoli
  Peanuts/peanut butter
  Yogurt
  Lentils

Pretzels
Pasta (white)
Graham crackers

Potatoes
Oat bran
Kidney beans

Grapes
Potato chips
Raisins/dried fruits

Black beans
Peaches
Ice cream

dairy products, leafy vegetables) and high fiber was shown to lower the risk of type 2 diabetes (Table 6.9). A diet that includes monounsaturated fats (e.g., olive oil, canola oil, nuts, and seeds) appears to lower LDL cholesterol while preserving HDL cholesterol levels.

In addition to promoting weight loss by creating a negative energy balance, exercise appears to have additional effects of specific importance to metabolic syndrome:
• Promote preferential loss of visceral fat
• Increase insulin sensitivity
• Improve plasma lipids
• Reduce blood pressure

The conditions that make up metabolic syndrome require pharmacologic management as well. Recommendations for medical management include the following. In the treatment of diabetes, consideration should be given to agents that don't promote weight gain, such as metformin (Glucophage) and the thiazolidinediones (Avandia, Actos). Lipid-lowering agents that lower triglycerides as well as total and LDL cholesterol, such as atorvastatin (Lipitor), are good choices. Blood pressure–lowering goals should be more ambitious in patients with both hypertension and diabetes. Current recommendations are that a target blood pressure of less than 130/85 mm Hg is appropriate.

Follow-up

When embarking on a weight loss program, patients should be seen monthly so the physician can assess progress and provide support. Patients with metabolic syndrome should be seen quarterly until they are meeting glycemic and blood pressure goals, and semiannually after that. At each visit, the physician should elicit information on lifestyle changes, adherence problems, and symptoms of complications. Physical examination should include checking blood pressure, weight, feet, pulses, sensation, and looking for any lesions. Glycosylated hemoglobin (Hgb A1c) should be checked quarterly until goals are met and then semiannually. A fasting lipid panel should be checked annually. Urinalysis should be performed annually to check for the presence of proteinuria and a measurement for microalbuminuria done if proteinuria is absent. Patients should be reminded of the importance of a yearly ophthalmologic exam. At each visit the management plan should be reviewed, including weight loss goals, dietary goals, exercise goals, and medication.

Patient Education

Patients should be encouraged to see this syndrome as one where they can make significant inroads with lifestyle changes. Patients can be told that weight loss need not be a huge amount. Many studies have shown that a mere 5% to 10% loss of initial weight can markedly improve many of these adverse risk factors.

Patients should be encouraged to take an active role in improving their health and to use the multitude of resources available in their community.

For physicians, an excellent resource is *Guidance for the Treatment of Adult Obesity,* 2nd ed. It can be ordered through Shape Up America!, 6707 Democracy Boulevard, Suite 306, Bethesda, MD 20817, or on the Web at http://www.shapeup.org.

SUGGESTED READINGS

Bray GA, Bouchard C, James WP. *Handbook of obesity.* New York: Marcel Dekker, 1998.

Carson JL, Ruddy ME, Duff AE, et al. The effect of gastric bypass surgery on hypertension in morbidly obese patients. *Arch Int Med* 1994;154:193.

Drenkowski A, Krahn DD, Demitrack L, et al. Naloxone, an opiate blocker, reduces the consumption of sweet, high fat foods in obese and lean female binge eaters. *Am J Clin Nutr* 1995;61:1206.

Fitzgibbon ML, Stolley MR, Kirshenbaum DS. Obese people who seek treatment are different than those who do not seek treatment. *Health Psychol* 1993;12:342.

Frohlich ED. Obesity and hypertension: converting enzyme inhibitors and calcium antagonists. *Hypertension* 1992;19[Suppl 1]:119.

Harris JK, French SA, Jeffrey RW, et al. Dietary and physical activity correlate of long-term weight loss. *Obes Res* 1994;2:307.

Jakicic JM, Wing RR, Butler P, et al. Prescribing exercise in multiple short bouts vs. one continuous bout: effects on adherence, cardiorespiratory fitness, and weight loss in overweight women. *Int J Obes Relat Metab Disord* 1995;19:893.

Jeffrey RW, Hellerstedt WL, French SA. A randomized trial of counseling for fat restriction vs. caloric restriction in the treatment of obesity. *Int J Obes Relat Metab Disord* 1995;19:132.

Kral JG. Surgical treatment of obesity. In: Bray GA, ed. *Handbook of obesity.* New York: Marcel Dekker, 1998.

Naslund I, Hallgren P, Sjostrom L. Fat cell weight and number before and after gastric surgery for morbid obesity in women. *Int J Obes Relat Metab Disord* 1988;12:191.

Pories WJ, Swanson MS, MacDonald KG, et al. Who would have thought it? An operation proves to be a more effective therapy for adult-onset diabetes mellitus. *Ann Surg* 1995;222:339.

Rand CS, MacGregor AM. Successful weight loss following obesity surgery and the perceived liability of morbid obesity. *Int J Obes Relat Metab Disord* 1991;15:577.

Schmeider RE, Gatzka C, Schachinger H, et al. Obesity as a determinant for the response to antihypertensive treatment. *Br Med J* 1993;307:537.

Serdula MK, Ivey D, Coates RJ, et al. Do obese children become obese adults? A review of the literature. *Prev Med* 1993;22:167.

Sjostrom L, William-Olsson T. Prospective studies on adipose development in men. *Int J Obes Relat Metab Disord* 1991;5:597.

CHAPTER 7

··

Depression and Other Mood Disorders

C. Carolyn Thiedke

DEPRESSION

Depression is a common mood disturbance, characterized by constitutional changes and physical and behavioral symptoms. It is seen more frequently among women than men. It is one of the most common disorders seen in a family physician's office. Recent research has led to a better understanding of depression as an illness with genetic and neurochemical roots but one that is affected by psychosocial factors as well.

Chief Complaints
- A 37-year-old mother of two presents to your office complaining of sadness, crying spells, increased irritability with her family, poor sleep, and poor appetite. She had a similar episode 7 years ago after the birth of her second child.
- A 73-year-old woman presents with her adult daughter and complains of feeling ill. The woman refuses to visit with friends or attend church the way she once did. She calls her family frequently to demand more attention to her complaints.

Clinical Manifestations
In its full-blown state, depression is easily recognized. The symptoms most familiar to family physicians can be found in Table 7.1. The challenge for many physicians is diagnosing depression when it presents in subsyndromic or atypical forms. Classification systems developed for psychiatrists may not be as useful in primary care settings, where patients' symptoms are more often undifferentiated.

T ABLE 7.1. Frequently encountered symptoms of depression

Emotional Changes	Behavioral Symptoms	Physical Symptoms	Cognitive Symptoms
Sad mood	Crying spells	Sleep disorder	Negative self-concept
Anxiety	Withdrawal	Eating disorder	Negative view of the world
Guilt	Agitation	Bowel disorder	Loss of hope for future
Anger	Retardation	Loss of energy	Self-blame
Diurnal mood variation	Hallucinations	Amenorrhea	Self-criticism
		Easy fatigue	Indecisiveness
		Weight change	Helplessness
		Decreased sex drive	Sense of worthlessness
		Pain	Delusions

Some simple questions to ask the patient when screening for depression include the following:
- Have you lost interest and pleasure in most things you usually enjoy?
- Have you lost energy or do you suffer from unexplained fatigue?
- Are you feeling sad, blue, or depressed?

Patients with depression may have a normal physical examination. However, some patients may display an affect that appears sad, anxious, or angry. Classically, patients with depression have been described as having psychomotor retardation—a dearth of the usual movements most people display when relating with someone. In severe depression, a woman's clothing or hair may appear disheveled.

Epidemiology

The National Institutes of Mental Health (NIMH) Epidemiological Catchment Area (ECA) survey calculated a prevalence of major depression in adults 18 years and older to be 5.0% and for dysthymia, a less severe but more chronic depression, 5.4%. Rates of all affective disorders were found to be higher in women (6.6%) than in men (3.5%). These disorders were more common among 25- to 44-year-olds and significantly less common in those greater than 65 years of age. The lifetime risk for a major depressive disorder is 20% to 25% in women.

Risk Factors

The incidence of depression is unrelated to race, education, income level, or citizenship status. Marital status can be a predictor of risk; women who are divorced or separated have higher risks of depression than those who are widowed or married. Other risk factors include the following:
- History of depressive illness
- First-degree relative with history of depressive illness
- Loss of parent before 10 years of age
- Childhood history of physical or sexual abuse
- Lack of social support
- Presence of a major social stressor or confluence of smaller social stressors
- Use of oral contraceptive with high progesterone content

Pathology

Explanations for depression have centered on five models:
- **Biologic model.** This model appears supported by the relationship of depression to hormonal change, the constancy of depression across cultures, the response of depression to medication and electroconvulsive therapy (ECT), and the evidence that certain medications cause depression. The strongest evidence suggests that depression stems from altered interplay of the many amines in the brain, predominantly norepinephrine and serotonin (or 5HT) and also dopamine.
- **Genetic model.** This model is based on the well-observed tendency for depression to run in families.
- **Psychoanalytic model.** This model associates depression with loss, failure, or rejection in childhood.
- **Cognitive model.** This credits the development of depression to cognitive distortions, such as automatic thoughts that keep people stuck in a negative view of the world.
- **Behavioral model.** This model suggests that the beginnings of depression occur in childhood when there is inadequate positive reinforcement for behaviors that promote healthy achievement.

Diagnosis

Depression can be an elusive diagnosis for family physicians. Certain conditions should prompt a physician to keep depression in mind (Table 7.2). If a physician suspects depression, he/she should also check the patient's medication list for medications that could be causing depression (Table 7.3).

Four patient-administered screening instruments have been tested in primary care settings:
- The General Health Questionnaire (GHQ), which has a subscale for depression
- The Center for Epidemiologic Studies—Depression Scale (CES-D)
- The Zung Self-Rating Depression Scale (ZSRDS)
- The Beck Depression Inventory (BDI)

T ABLE 7.2.   Medical conditions that can lead to depression

Cerebrovascular accident
Dementia, including Alzheimer's
Diabetes
Coronary artery disease
Cancer
Chronic fatigue syndrome
Fibromyalgia

T ABLE 7.3.   Medications that have been associated with depression

Cardiovascular drugs	Hormones
Methyldopa (Aldomet)	Oral contraceptives
Reserpine (Serpasil)	Glucocorticoids
Propranolol (Inderal)	Anabolic steroids
Clonidine (Catapres)	
Thiazide diuretics	Psychotropics
Digoxin (Lanoxin)	Benzodiazepines
	Neuroleptics
Anticancer agents	
Cycloserine (Seromycin)	Others
	Cocaine
Anti-inflammatory/anti-infective agents	Amphetamines
NSAIDs	L-dopa
Ethambutol (Myambutol)	Cimetidine (Tagamet), ranitidine (Zantac)
Disulfiram (Antabuse)	
Sulfonamides	
Baclofen (Lioresal)	
Metoclopramide (Reglan)	

These instruments produce few false-negative results, but they have false-positive rates of 25% to 40%. Thus, although they detect all patients who have major depression, they also identify many who ultimately prove not to have a mood disorder. To improve the positive predictive value of these screening tests, it is wise to limit their use to patients who are at high risk for depression:

- Patients with chronic disease
- Patients with unexplained or ill-defined symptoms
- Patients with sleep complaints
- Patients with a history of psychiatric illness
- Patients with headaches, abdominal pain, or other pain syndromes
- Patients with unexplained fatigue
- Patients with either a sad mood or professed anhedonia

Depression may present differently in women and men. Recognizing these differences may assist a physician in making the diagnosis (Table 7.4).

No completely reliable diagnostic tests is available for depression. However, in women greater than 50 years of age with symptoms of depression, thyroid function tests should be done to rule out undiagnosed hypothyroidism.

Referral

A family physician may wish to refer a patient in the following circumstances:

- Lack of response to an adequate trial with one or more antidepressants
- An opinion regarding the usefulness of psychotherapy for a particular patient
- Diagnostic uncertainty
- Severe, recurrent, or psychotic depression
- Need for ECT
- Need for hospitalization
- Need for involuntary commitment
- Suicidal risk
- Significant medical or psychiatric comorbidities

Management

Before the advent of modern psychopharmacology, psychotherapy was the treatment of choice for depression. Today many medications are available that have proved effective in the treatment of depression. No one medication has been shown to be more effective than others and no single medication provides remission for all patients. The medication selected is based on the following factors:

- Side-effect profile
- Patient history of prior response

T ABLE 7.4. Female-specific assessment of depression

Look for atypical symptoms, more symptoms, greater comorbidity in women
Look for different patterns of comorbidity
Assess course features: longer episodes, more chronic and recurrent illness in women
Look for triggers of episodes: stressful life events, seasonal pattern, reproductive events
Look for premenstrual exacerbations of illness
Assess psychosocial factors (e.g., victimization, role stress)

Adapted from Kornstein S. Gender differences in depression: implications for treatment. *J Clin Psychiatr* 1997;58 [Suppl 15]:12.

- Family history of response
- Type of depression
- Cost
- Physician familiarity and comfort with medication
- Frequency of administration (ease of administration, impact on patient lifestyle)
- Patient preference
    Medications have several clear benefits over psychotherapy:
- Ease of administration
- Efficacy
- Little requirement of patient time
- Widely available
    Medications have some disadvantages, however:
- Need for repeated office visits to practitioner, at least initially, to monitor response and need for dosage adjustments
- Side effects
- Potential use in suicide attempt
- Failure of patients to continue medications
- Occasional lack of efficacy
- Need for patient compliance with medication schedule
- Need for ongoing evaluation for long-term use
    Medication should be initiated with or without psychotherapy for patients with the following factors:
- Moderate to severe depression
- Chronic, recurrent, psychotic, or melancholic depression
- Prior positive response to medication for depression
- Family history
- Patient preference
- Failure to respond to psychotherapy alone
    Table 7.5 lists medications commonly used to treat depression.
    Psychotherapy alone continues to be a treatment option today in mild depression. Psychotherapy has some advantages over medication in the treatment of depression:
- Psychotherapy does not cause physiologic side effects common with pharmacologic agents.
- Some patients may respond to therapy when medications have not proved effective (not empirically documented).
- Because psychotherapy teaches patients to alter lifestyle factors that may lead to depression, it may theoretically lessen the chance of recurrences (evidence is inconclusive).
    Psychotherapy, however, has several disadvantages when compared with medication:
- It has rarely been tested in patients with severe or psychotic depression.
- Ten percent to 40% of patients fail to complete a full course of therapy.
- Many forms of time-limited psychotherapy have not been tested by randomized, controlled clinical trials.
- Therapy sessions may be time-consuming and inconvenient.
- Outcomes are related to the skill of the therapist.
- Skilled therapists may not be widely available.
- The cost of long-term psychotherapy may be high and may not be covered by insurance.
- It takes longer to see the benefit of treatment (6 to 8 weeks) than it does with medication (4 to 6 weeks).

T ABLE 7.5. Medications used in the treatment of depression

Drug (Trade Name)	Therapeutic Range (mg/day)	Side-effect Profile
Tricyclics		
Amitriptyline (Elavil)	75–300	a,b,c,d,e,g
Desipramine (Norpramin)	75–300	a,b,c,d,e
Doxepin (Sinequan)	75–300	a,b,c,d,e,g
Imipramine (Tofranil)	75–300	a,b,c,d,e,g
Nortriptyline (Pamelor)	40–150	d,e
Protriptyline (Vivactil)	20–60	a,c,d,e
Trimipramine (Surmontil)	75–300	a,b,c,e,g
Heterocyclics		
Amoxapine (Asendin)	100–600	a,b,c,d,e,g
Bupropion (Wellbutrin)	225–450	c
Maprotiline (Ludiomil)	100–225	a,b,c,d,e,g
Trazodone (Desyrel)	150–600	b,g
Venlafaxine (Effexor)	75–375	b,f,g
SSRIs		
Fluoxetine (Prozac)	10–40	c,f
Paroxetine (Paxil)	20–50	c,f
Sertraline (Zoloft)	50–150	c,f
Citalopram (Celexa)	10–40	c,d,f
MAOIs		
Isocarboxazid (Marplan)	10–40	c,d,g
Phenelzine (Nardil)	15–90	b,c,d,g
Tranylcypromine (Parnate)	20–60	c,d,g

Abbreviations: a, anticholinergic; b, drowsiness; c, insomnia; d, orthostatic hypotension; e, cardiac arrhythmias; f, gastrointestinal distress; g, weight gain.

The combination of medication and psychotherapy is also an option. Some authors recommend that it be reserved until a trial with each alone has proved partially effective. Initial combination therapy has the disadvantages of the individual components and makes it difficult to evaluate which modality was the most efficacious. (This is important information for the treatment of future recurrences.) Combination therapy may be helpful when there are different desired outcomes (e.g., symptom relief from medication and marital, social, and psychologic benefits from therapy). It may also be helpful in chronic depression when quality of life remains poor.

Several forms of psychotherapy have been studied for efficacy:
- Cognitive therapy teaches patients to become aware of and counteract their distorted, negative, moment-to-moment thinking.
- Behavioral therapy teaches patients specific behaviors, such as activity scheduling, self-control, problem solving, and social skills.
- Interpersonal therapy helps patients resolve issues such as role disputes, social isolation, prolonged grief reaction, and role transition.
- Marital therapy.

- Brief dynamic therapy uses traditional techniques of examining core conflicts, but in a time-limited fashion.

Many therapists use a variety of approaches in the same patient, depending on her needs. Thus a patient may be instructed in cognitive behavior therapy while exploring interpersonal issues and having joint sessions for marital therapy with her spouse.

Research examining the effectiveness of all these psychotherapies has found that study subjects receiving therapy improved, compared with controls who were on waiting lists to be seen. When compared with pharmacotherapy for mild to moderate depression, these therapies have been found to be equally efficacious in the acute stage (approximately 50% response rate). The overall efficacy of group therapy appears to be somewhat less than that of individual therapy (39% versus 50%).

Electroconvulsive Therapy

Although family physicians do not perform ECT, they may feel a patient is a candidate for it and therefore select a referral psychiatrist with expertise in its use. ECT, which is the use of electrically-induced repetitive firings of the neurons in the central nervous system, was first discovered to be beneficial in the treatment of depression in the late 1930s. It continues to be an option for certain types of patients today and should be considered in patients with the following factors:
- Severe major depressive disorder that has not responded to adequate trials of antidepressant medications
- Psychotic depression
- Medical risk posed by antidepressant or neuroleptic medications
- Psychomotor retardation, suicidal risk, or other condition that requires a rapid improvement in symptoms
- Previous response to ECT
- Mixed manic episodes
- Schizoaffective disorder responding only partially to medication
- Catatonia
- Melancholic symptoms that have previously failed to respond to medications

Studies of ECT with controls who receive a simulated procedure find it to be highly effective in inpatients with severe depression. It may not be as effective in less severe depression.

Typically, patients in the United States receive treatments every other day for 2 to 3 weeks. The number of treatments administered is determined by the patient's response. A course of six to 10 treatments is typical. ECT is a safe procedure, with risks not significantly greater than the anesthesia given before the treatment. The most frequent complaints by patients after the procedure are memory impairment, headaches, and muscle aches.

Exercise

Exercise was shown in one study to be as effective as psychotherapy in mild to moderate depression. An exercise prescription might therefore be a useful adjunct to medication.

Light Therapy

Light therapy has proved effective in patients with seasonal affective disorder. Morning exposure to bright light appears to provide the best results. Light boxes can be purchased from sources on the Internet that provide the currently recommended 2,500 lux for 2 hours each day for a week. Doses as high as 10,000 lux for briefer periods of time may prove to be even more beneficial. Light therapy can be used in combination with medication.

St. John's Wort

A metaanalysis of 23 randomized or quasirandomized controlled trials found that St. John's wort has a rate of effectiveness of 60% to 70% in the treatment of mild to moderate depression. Recommendations for dosing are 900 mg/day in three divided doses. This herbal remedy is generally well tolerated, with a more favorable side-effect profile than the tricyclics. The most commonly noted side effects are nausea and dizziness. Patients should be warned about photosensitivity. There is the possibility of interaction with monamine oxidase and serotonin, so St. John's wort should not be used along with monoamine oxidase inhibitors (MAOIs) or selective serotonin reuptake inhibitors (SSRIs).

Counseling

Counseling by the primary care physician as a form of therapy has not been well studied, although it occurs regularly. One study of British general practitioners trained to use a problem-solving technique found a response rate equivalent to medication. Most family physicians intuitively dispense helpful guidance in conjunction with medication. Giving patients homework to do between visits, such as keeping a diary of symptoms, trying new behaviors, reaching out socially, or being more assertive, encourages patients to become "unstuck" and helps provide structure for follow-up visits.

Family physicians may certainly employ many of the techniques used by therapists to help the patient get better. The BATHE technique is encouraged as a means of discussing psychosocial issues so they fit within the framework of the family physician's typical 15-minute office visit. BATHE is an acronym:

- **B** = *Background.* "What's going on in your life?"
- **A** = *Affect.* "How do you feel about that?" or "What is your mood?"
- **T** = *Trouble.* "What about the situation troubles you the most?"
- **H** = *Handling.* "How are you handling that?"
- **E** = *Empathy.* "That must be very difficult for you."

Often just being BATHE'd is therapeutic, as the patient feels she has been listened to and understood. Frequently, however, the process suggests areas where the patient can do homework before the next visit.

Follow-up

Clinical practice guidelines for the diagnosis and treatment of depression have been developed by an expert panel after a systematic review of the research literature in conjunction with the Agency for Healthcare Research and Quality (AHRQ). They recommend that patients with severe depression be seen weekly for the first 6 to 8 weeks of treatment and then every 4 to 12 weeks when the depression has largely resolved. Patients whose depression is less severe may be seen every 10 to 14 days for the first 6 to 8 weeks.

If a patient has not responded to medication in the first 6 weeks of treatment, the diagnosis should be reassessed. If it is still believed that depression is the correct diagnosis, the following interventions may be appropriate:

- Increase the dosage of medication
- Change to another antidepressant
- Add a second medication (this is a less preferred intervention, according to the AHRQ guidelines)
- Refer the patient for psychotherapy

If there has been a partial response, medication can be continued at the current dose and the patient can either be reevaluated in another 6 weeks or be referred for psychotherapy. If there has been no response at that point, the medication should be increased or changed, or referral to a psychiatrist should be considered.

See Figs. 7.1, 7.2, and 7.3 for suggested algorithms for follow-up.

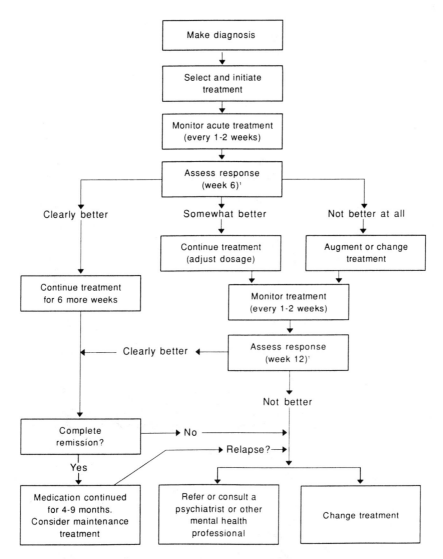

¹Times of assessment (weeks 6 and 12) rest on very modest data. It may be necessary to revise the treatment plan earlier for patients failing to respond at all.

FIGURE 7.1. Overview of treatment for depression. (Reproduced from Depression Guideline Panel. *Depression in primary care.* Vol 2: *Treatment of major depression.* Clinical Practice Guideline No. 5. Rockville, MD: U.S. Department of Health and Human Services, Public Health Service, Agency for Health Care Policy and Research. AHCPR Publication No. 93-0551. April 1993.)

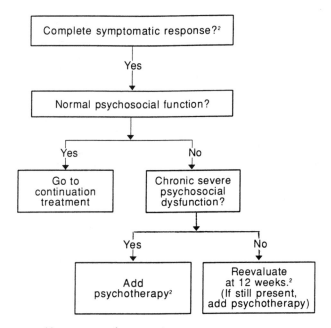

Complete response—with no or very few symptoms.
[2]These suggestions are based on indirectly relevant data, logical inference, and clinical experience.

FIGURE 7.2. Six-week evaluation: responders to medication. (Reproduced from Depression Guideline Panel. *Depression in primary care.* Vol 2: *Treatment of major depression.* Clinical Practice Guideline No. 5. Rockville, MD: U.S. Department of Health and Human Services, Public Health Service, Agency for Health Care Policy and Research. AHCPR Publication No. 93-0551. April 1993.)

To prevent relapse, it is recommended that once the patient has reached stability on a certain dosage of medication, the medication should be continued at that dosage for 4 (for those in whom the onset of depression is clearly known) and possibly 9 months (for those in whom depression has lasted 2 or more years). Certain patients should be considered for long-term maintenance therapy:
1. Those with three or more episodes of major depressive disorder
2. Those with two episodes of major depressive disorder and the following:
   a. Family history of bipolar disorder
   b. Recurrence of depression within 1 year of a successfully treated episode
   c. Family history of recurrent major depressive disorder
   d. Onset of depression before age 20
   e. Both episodes were severe, sudden, and life-threatening, and occurred within 3 years

Discontinuing Medications
Tricyclic antidepressants (TCAs) need to be tapered over 2 to 4 weeks. There is no evidence that bupropion (Wellbutrin), MAOIs, fluoxetine (Prozac), paroxetine (Paxil), sertraline (Zoloft), or trazodone (Desyrel) must be tapered.

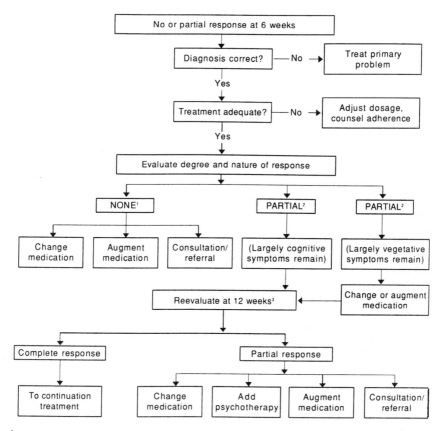

[^1]: No response—patient is nearly as symptomatic as at pretreatment.
[^2]: Partial response—patient is clearly better than at pretreatment, but still has significant symptoms. Consultation or referral may be valuable before proceeding further.
[^3]: Suggestions for management are based on some indirectly relevant studies. logic, and clinical experience.

FIGURE 7.3. Six-week evaluation: partial responders or nonresponders to medication. (Reproduced from Depression Guideline Panel. *Depression in primary care.* Vol 2: *Treatment of major depression.* Clinical Practice Guideline No. 5. Rockville, MD: U.S. Department of Health and Human Services, Public Health Service, Agency for Health Care Policy and Research. AHCPR Publication No. 93-0551. April 1993.)

It is important that patients be informed about the possibility of a recurrence of symptoms either during maintenance treatment or after the medication has been discontinued. They should be instructed to contact their physicians if they experience a return of their symptoms.

Suicide

Suicide is the most tragic complication of depression. Women attempt suicide more frequently but are less often successful than men. The following are thought to be risk factors for suicide:

- Feelings of hopelessness
- General medical illnesses
- Family history of substance abuse
- Substance abuse
- Caucasian
- Psychotic symptoms
- Living alone
- Prior suicide attempts
- Having a specific, realistic, plan
- Having a gun

Physicians should assess suicidal risk during their initial interview with depressed patients by asking directly about suicidal ideation. A physician may ask, "Have you considered harming yourself?" If the patient indicates she has, then the physician should ask:

- How seriously have you considered suicide?
- Have you taken any steps to carry out your plan?
- Have you taken any steps to prepare for your death?
- Have you ever tried to harm yourself before?
- Do you ever abuse alcohol or drugs?
- What would keep you from attempting suicide?
- Who do you have to support you?
- Will you agree to call me or another support person if you feel like harming yourself?

If the risk of suicide seems high, the patient should be hospitalized. If the situation is not critical, the patient may be treated on an outpatient basis, but the physician is encouraged to take the following steps:

- Provide hope for the patient by discussing the successful treatment of depression
- Develop a contract in which the patient agrees to notify the physician if suicidal feelings become stronger
- Be readily available to the patient
- Strongly encourage the patient to abstain from alcohol and drugs
- See the patient weekly while suicidal ideation is present
- Provide only one week's worth of medications
- Attempt to bolster social support for the patient
- Advise the patient to remove instruments of suicide from her home

Patient Education

In addition to prescribing medications, family physicians can provide comfort to depressed patients by the following means:

- Establish a relationship of trust and caring
- Strengthen hope
- Set realistic goals
- Provide education about the nature of the illness
- Provide a plan for relief of symptoms
- Discourage major life changes during the depressed episode or for a time afterward
- Enlist the support of significant others in the patient's life
- Celebrate successful experiences with the patient
- Be vigilant for the appearance of suicidal impulses

Physicians have the twin responsibilities of emphasizing the treatable nature of depression and at the same time warning about the likelihood of recurrence, particularly if medication or therapy is ended prematurely.

PREMENSTRUAL DYSPHORIC DISORDER

Premenstrual dysphoric disorder (PMDD) is a cyclically occurring mood disorder associated with the luteal, or premenstrual, phase of a woman's hormonal cycle. PMDD is present in a subset of patients who have premenstrual syndrome (PMS). These women have mood-related symptoms that can be severe and debilitating at times.

Chief Complaint

- A 38-year-old woman presents complaining of symptoms that sometimes seem unmanageable. She becomes enraged by circumstances that she can handle at other times with equanimity. She feels down during these periods and feels she can barely get through her day. She notices these symptoms during the week before her menses.

Clinical Manifestations

To meet the criteria for PMDD, a woman should experience five or more of the following symptoms during the last week of her luteal phase (adapted from DSM-IV): markedly depressed mood, marked anxiety, marked affective lability, persistent anger or irritability, decreased interest in usual activities, subjective sense of difficulty in concentrating, lethargy, marked change in appetite, hypersomnia or insomnia, subjective sense of being overwhelmed or out of control, physical symptoms such as breast tenderness, headaches, joint or muscle pain, bloating sensation, or weight gain. The symptoms should largely remit within a few days of the follicular phase and be absent for at least a week after menses.

Epidemiology

Recent reviews of epidemiologic studies reveal that 80% of women experience mild to moderate premenstrual symptoms at some point during their fertile years. It appears that 3% to 8% of women experience symptoms severe enough to be considered disabling. Prospective studies using symptom diaries confirm this prevalence of 3% to 8%.

Risk Factors

- Comorbidity with major depressive disorder is high. Estimates range from 30% to 80%.
- Comorbidity exists with bipolar effective disorder, but the diagnoses are often difficult to distinguish because both involve cycling of symptoms.
- Not surprisingly, there is also a high comorbidity with generalized anxiety disorder, social phobia, and panic attacks.

Pathology

The cause of this disorder has been elusive despite considerable research effort examining hormonal fluctuations, thyroid hormone levels, prostaglandin levels, and insulin levels. Several studies have pointed to a decline in beta endorphins in symptomatic women when compared with control subjects. The studies have varied, however, in methodology, patient selection, and size. Other studies have found changes in adrenergic activity and gamma-aminobutyric acid (GABA) levels. The bulk of the evidence is related to serotonin (or 5HT) and its precursor, tryptophan.

Diagnosis

Diagnosis of PMDD is made by history alone. There are no physical findings or diagnostic tests that are useful. To distinguish PMDD from major depressive disorder, dysthymia, anxiety disorder, or bipolar disorder, a careful symptom diary must be kept by the patient for at least two menstrual cycles. Only then can it become determined whether symptoms cluster during the luteal phase and remit for at least 1 week after menses.

Referral

Once the diagnosis has been made, a woman's family physician can work with her to improve her symptoms. If the depressive symptoms are particularly severe and do not respond to medication, referral to a psychiatrist may be considered.

Management

Trials using several antidepressants, such as clomipramine (Anafranil), bupropion (Wellbutrin), maprotiline (Ludiomil), sertraline (Zoloft), and venlafaxine (Effexor) have found that these agents are effective when compared with placebo.

However, the greatest weight of evidence of effectiveness lies with the SSRIs, fluoxetine (Prozac), and paroxetine (Paxil). Citalopram (Celexa) has shown benefit over placebo in a controlled study. Other treatments (not all FDA approved for this indication) include:

- Alprazolam (Xanax) given during the luteal phase was found to be superior to placebo.
- Another study found that propranolol (Inderal) 20 mg/day (40 mg during menses) lowered symptoms by 59%.
- Recent trials using calcium at 1,200 mg elemental calcium/day found a reduction in symptoms by 60%.
- Gonadotrophin-releasing hormone (GnRH) agonists have also been found to be effective, but they can cause menopausal symptoms and should therefore be reserved for women whose symptoms resist other forms of therapy.
- Results have been inconsistent with hormonal treatment, including estrogen and synthetic progestins. Anecdotal reports of the benefits of natural progesterone exist but have not been studied in controlled trials with larger numbers of patients.
- Cognitive behavior therapy and group therapy have been shown to reduce symptom severity in some women with PMDD.

Traditionally, women with PMDD or PMS have been given the following advice regarding lifestyle changes:
- Increased aerobic activity
- Reduced caffeine intake
- Reduced alcohol intake
- Less dietary fat and refined carbohydrates and more complex carbohydrates (e.g., whole grain products and legumes)
- Some form of relaxation therapy

The evidence for the effectiveness of these interventions is sketchy, but they may still be recommended because they are, in general, health-promoting behaviors and may provide women with the sense that they can control or lessen their symptoms.

Follow-up

Until a woman's symptoms are well controlled, she should be seen monthly. Once her symptoms are well controlled, symptom relief has been achieved, and she remains comfortable with her therapy, she can be seen every 6 to 12 months until menopause.

Patient Education

As with other mood disorders, a physician may offer a woman a sense of hope about the treatable nature of this condition. She should be told that her symptoms will likely remit after menopause, but until then, she should continue whatever lifestyle or other treatment measures bring relief. It is important to stress that the root of this condition is probably biologic rather than emotional or characterologic.

POSTPARTUM DEPRESSION

No other life event rivals pregnancy and childbirth in terms of neuroendocrine fluctuations and psychosocial effects. Postpartum mood disorders affect a significant number of new mothers.

Chief Complaint

- You receive a call from the husband of one of your patients who delivered her first child 3 weeks ago. He notes that she seems drained of life. She has stopped bathing and eating, and seems withdrawn from him. She appears not to tolerate the cries of her infant and often dissolves into tears herself.

Clinical Manifestations

Postpartum depression is characterized by the following symptoms that appear within 6 weeks of giving birth:
- Mood lability
- Tearfulness
- Anxiety
- Irritability
- Appetite and sleep disturbances

Epidemiology

DSM-IV now includes a category of postpartum mood disorders. The three major subtypes include the following:
- Maternity "blues"
- Postpartum major depression
- Postpartum psychosis

Researchers are also beginning to look at the postpartum period as a time for the onset of obsessive-compulsive disorder (OCD) and panic disorder. Maternity blues are common and mild, generally affecting up to 85% of new mothers at some time during the first 2 weeks after the birth of a child. Approximately 10% to 20% of these women will go on to develop postpartum major depression. For 60% of these women, it will be their first bout of depression. The prevalence of postpartum depression is somewhat higher in adolescent mothers, approximately 26%.

Postpartum psychosis is a rare condition that affects one to two mothers per 1,000 live births. This can be a severe psychosis and often represents a bipolar disorder or a unipolar depression with psychotic features.

Risk Factors

A personal or family history of depression puts one at greater risk of postpartum depression. A woman with a previous history of postpartum depression has a 50% risk of developing postpartum depression with subsequent pregnancies. Anxiety or depression during pregnancy puts a woman at greater risk. Other proposed risk factors include the following:
- Poor postpartum support
- Stressful or adverse life circumstances
- Marital instability
- An infant that is hard to soothe or demands extra care
- Undesired pregnancy

Pathology

Hormonal theories as to the etiology of postpartum depression seem logical, but thus far no studies looking at various neuroendocrine systems have shown a difference between women with and women without postpartum depression. One theory focuses on thyroid dysfunction and the hypothalamic-pituitary-thyroid (HPT) axis. A follow-up study of women who displayed antithyroid antibodies at 16 weeks' gestation found a 50% chance of postpartum depression. The mechanism by which the HPT axis may be involved in postpartum depression remains obscure.

Diagnosis

Postpartum depression is a diagnosis based on history. The challenge is separating the normal feelings of the "baby blues" from true postpartum depression. Psychologic complaints that persist after the first 2 weeks, and are separated by more than 3 days, should alert the physician to explore further for postpartum depression.

There are no specific diagnostic tests that are helpful in diagnosing postpartum depression, although thyroid dysfunction should be considered and tested for if other signs or symptoms suggest it.

Referral

Many patients whose symptoms are mild can be managed with reassurance and extra support. Family physicians may also feel comfortable prescribing antidepressants for these patients. Patients who may be suicidal, who are psychotic, or who may desire ECT rather than pharmacologic treatment should be referred to a psychiatrist.

Management

For mothers who are not breastfeeding, the range of antidepressant options is the same as that for women who are not post partum. Historically, both physicians and nursing mothers have been concerned about the effects of antidepressants on infants. Some medications have been studied, however, and have been found to be effective, with no reported adverse effects in infants. However, long-term studies of effects on infants who are breastfed while their mothers take these medications are not available. Medications that have been studied include the following:

* Clomipramine (Anafranil)
* Amitriptyline (Elavil)
* Imipramine (Tofranil)
* Desipramine (Norpramin)
* Nortriptyline (Pamelor)
* Bupropion (Wellbutrin)
* Sertraline (Zoloft)

Psychotherapeutic interventions have also been shown to reduce symptoms in a group setting over 12 weeks.

Measures to help support the new mother, although not studied, seem logical. Enlisting the spouse, family, friends, or even outside help will lighten the new mother's feeling of being burdened and overwhelmed. Other health measures, such as exercise, healthy eating, and sufficient rest, may be suggested.

Patient Education

As with the other mood disorders, the treatable nature of this disorder should be emphasized to the patient and her spouse. It is critical that the woman be told that the presence of postpartum depression in no way reflects on her worth or competence as a mother. She should be reassured that infants are quite resilient and that her depression will leave no lasting effects on her child. She should be told that she may be at risk for depression with or without subsequent pregnancies and that she should be alert for symptoms and see her physician should they develop.

SUGGESTED READINGS

American Psychiatric Association. *Diagnostic and statistical manual of mental disorders,* 4th ed. Primary care version. Washington, DC: APA, 1995.

Bhatia SC, Bhatia SK. Depression in women: diagnostic and treatment considerations. *Am Fam Physician* 1999;60:225.

Depression in primary care, vol 1: *Detection and diagnosis.* Clinical Practice Guideline No. 5. Rockville, MD: U.S. Department of Health and Human Services, Public Health Service, Agency for Health Care Policy and Research, 1993.

Depression in primary care, vol 2. *Treatment of major depression.* Clinical Practice Guideline No. 5. Rockville, MD: U.S. Department of Health and Human Services, Public Health Service, Agency for Health Care Policy and Research, 1993.

Kornstein SG. Gender differences in depression: implications for treatment. *J Clin Psychiatry* 1997;58[Suppl 15]:12.

Llewellyn AM, Stowe ZN, Nemeroff CB. Depression during pregnancy and the puerperium. *J Clin Psychiatry* 1997;58[Suppl 15]:26.

Schuyler D. *Taming the tyrant: treating depressed adults.* New York; Norton, 1998.

Stuart M, Lieberman J. *The fifteen minute hour: applied psychotherapy for the primary care physician,* 2nd ed. Westport, CT: Praeger, 1993.

Yonkers KA. The association between premenstrual dysphoric disorder and other mood disorders. *J Clin Psychiatry* 1997;58[Suppl 15]:19.

CHAPTER 8

....

Sexual Issues for Women

C. Carolyn Thiedke

Sexual problems have been found to be exceedingly common when various populations have been surveyed. Those same surveys have generally found that patients are grateful when a discussion of sexual matters is initiated by their physicians. Yet many physicians have not incorporated questions regarding sexual function into their routine history taking.

A few basic questions can be incorporated into the medical history. Asked in a straightforward and low-key manner, they are likely to be well accepted by patients (Table 8.1). If problems are discovered, a more in-depth history can be obtained (Table 8.2). This line of questioning takes more time, and the patient can be asked to return for another visit so that problems can be dealt with in greater depth.

Physicians should be aware that sexual issues are difficult for patients to discuss and may present covertly. Be sensitive to behavior that does not "fit"—for example, the patient who complains of discharge when there is little, is concerned about an odor when you find none, or has had multiple partners yet seems fearful of the physical examination. An awareness of our own confusion as physicians about what is going on can be an effective diagnostic tool. Speaking of it to patients may open the door to a frank discussion of a troubling matter, often sexual abuse, that has been hidden.

When examining sexual dysfunction, it is helpful first to outline normal human sexual response. Doing so gives physicians a schema for understanding where problems can arise. The first phase is desire to engage in sex. This is followed by arousal if a partner is present or the patient masturbates, orgasm, and resolution. Dysfunction in the arousal stage can be caused by hypoactive sexual desire disorder or sexual aver-

---

T ABLE 8.1. The basic sexual history for routine visits

1. Have you noticed any problems in your ability to have and enjoy sex?
2. Do you have any pain during penetration?
3. Do you have any difficulty having an orgasm?
4. Are you currently sexually active? Do you have sex with men, women, or both?
5. Do you have any questions or concerns about your sexual functioning?

Any positive responses should be followed up by attempts to further clarify the problem:

1. How much of a problem is this?
2. How long has this been a problem? When was it better or worse?
3. Do you have any ideas about what causes the problem?
4. Have you ever sought help for this problem before?
5. How do you feel about getting some help now?

T ABLE 8.2. Detailed sexual history

History of the presenting problem	Masturbatory practices
Time of onset	Homosexual experiences
Mode of onset	Past history of negative sexual experiences
Duration	Family history
Situational context	Family of origin attitudes toward sexuality
Exacerbations and remissions	Parents' sexuality
Effect of any attempted management	Religious beliefs about sexuality
Associated symptoms	Current relationship with family of origin
Current sexual relationship	Family violence
Frequency of sex	Relationship history
Frequency both partners would prefer	History and stability of current relationship
Time of day of lovemaking	Changes in feelings toward partner
Presence of fatigue	Presence of unresolved conflict
Problems with privacy	Infidelity
Communication of desire, verbal and nonverbal	Communication problems
What constitutes foreplay	Current stressors
Level of arousal	Within the family
Frequency of orgasm	Outside the family
Cognitive activities that occur during sex	Family life cycle issues
Pain	Medical history
Contraceptive	Acute illness
Paraphilias	Chronic illness
Sexual history	Injuries
Early experiences	Surgery
Puberty	Medications
Attitudes toward sexuality	Substance abuse
Level of sexual knowledge	Review of systems
Extent of previous sexual experience	
Ascription to cultural sexual myths	

sion. In the excitement phase, dysfunction can be caused by dyspareunia from several sources and female sexual arousal disorder. Problems in the orgasmic phase can be from inhibited orgasm or anorgasmia. This chapter will deal with several of these concerns.

When addressing sexual problems, family physicians should not assume that all women are engaged in marital or heterosexual relationships. When possible, it is advisable to use language that is inclusive and does not make these assumptions.

HYPOACTIVE SEXUAL DESIRE DISORDER

Hypoactive sexual desire disorder (HSDD) is a common but frequently undiagnosed concern in women. However, the media attention given to sildenafil (Viagra) in the late 1990s may change that. Sexual dysfunction as an issue for discussion between physicians and patients has been given legitimacy, and women may therefore feel freer to bring this concern up during office visits.

Chief Complaint

- A 43-year-old patient whom you have known for several years and with whom you have a strong relationship mentions during her physical that she has lost interest in sex. She feels that neither her relationship with her husband nor their style of lovemaking has significantly changed.

Clinical Manifestations

By definition, HSDD displays itself as persistently low or absent level of sexual fantasies or desire for sexual activity. To be classified as HSDD, medical causes, substance abuse, or other Axis I diagnoses must be ruled out. Distinction must be made between primary and secondary HSDD. In primary HSDD the following are generally found:
- Sexual fantasies are absent
- Masturbation occurs infrequently
- The woman has generally had limited sexual experience, with few partners
- She feels little or no pleasure in sensual exchange
- These characteristics have persisted since childhood

In secondary HSDD the patient acknowledges the following:
- An early period of active desire and sexual involvement
- An interest in fantasy and masturbation
- Attraction to other partners

During the physical examination, the physician should look for signs of chronic systemic illness. In addition, the signs of endocrine disturbances (e.g., diabetes, thyroid, adrenal, or pituitary dysfunction) must be assessed. The presence or absence of secondary sex characteristics is an important diagnostic point.

Epidemiology

Surveys have shown that sexual problems occur in 50% of all marriages, and 75% of couples who seek marital counseling have a sexual complaint. Moore and Goldstein found that 56% of patients in a family practice setting reported at least one sexual concern. Frank's survey of well-adjusted couples found that 77% reported "sexual difficulties."

In a large-scale study of the full spectrum of sexual dysfunction, 65% of respondents had primary HSDD (81% of whom were women). A large overlap was found between HSDD and other types of sexual dysfunction. Forty percent of patients with HSDD also had diagnoses of arousal or orgasmic disorder.

Risk Factors

In the presence of the competing emotions of anxiety and anger, women show a greater decline than men in sexual interest. In one study of the survivors of sexual abuse, 85% had subsequent sexual arousal or desire difficulties. Career women were more likely to report HSDD than women in less demanding jobs or women who were not employed outside the home. Younger women, whose relationships tend to be more unstable, had higher levels of sexual dysfunction than older women. African-American women had higher rates of HSDD but were less likely to experience pain with intercourse. A falling income was strongly associated with sexual disinterest in women. Anything that causes marital dissatisfaction may manifest itself as HSDD (Table 8.3). Any congenital or acquired condition that affects sexual anatomy can put a woman at risk for HSDD. Women who are hypoandrogenic either from hysterectomy, bilateral salpingo-oophorectomy, or cancer chemotherapy are at risk for HSDD. It is known that

T ABLE 8.3. Causes of relationship discord

Poor communication
Unrealistic expectations
Failure to resolve conflicts
Loss of trust
Fear of intimacy
Poor relationship modeling by parents
Family system distress (e.g., teenager acting out; care of elderly parent)
Conflicts about sex roles
Divergent sexual preferences or values
Career problems
Demands of household and child care
Financial difficulties
Legal problems

there are testosterone receptors in the female brain, and the absence of testosterone leads to a diminished desire, decreased sensitivity of the clitoris and nipples to stimulation, decreased muscle tone, and decreased arousal and capacity for orgasm.

Diagnosis

Several conditions can affect sexual functioning that should be considered before diagnosing HSDD:
• Chronic illness
• Pregnancy
• Pharmacologic agents (Table 8.4)
• Endocrine alterations (e.g., thyroid, diabetes, hyperprolactinemia)
• Chemical substance abuse
   A high comorbidity is found between HSDD and depression, anxiety, and somatic complaints. Seventy-one percent of patients with HSDD give a history consistent with a lifetime diagnosis of affective disorder.

Diagnostic Testing

In comparisons of eugonadal women with HSDD and control subjects, no differences in testosterone, estradiol, progesterone, or prolactin levels were found. Screening for chronic illness or endocrine abnormalities can be accomplished with a complete blood count (CBC), fasting glucose, urinalysis, thyroid stimulating hormone (TSH), liver function tests, and a blood urea nitrogen (BUN) and creatinine level. A prolactin level can be checked if there is other evidence to suggest an abnormality.

Referral

Physicians are encouraged to become comfortable providing care for sexual issues. Practice at broaching these issues and working through them with patients leads to greater satisfaction and attainment of skill, similar to the acquisition of any medical procedure. As stated by Stuart and Lieberman in *The Fifteen Minute Hour,* family physicians should attempt to treat patients, where possible, rather than refer them, for the following reasons:
• Referrals made are often not kept.

T ABLE 8.4. Commonly prescribed agents that have been reported to cause decreased sexual desire

Antihypertensives	Protriptyline (Vivactil)
Amiloride (Midamor)	Other psychotropic medications
Benazepril (Lotensin)	Most benzodiazepines
Clonidine (Catapres)	Barbiturates
Chlorthalidone (Hygroton)	Buspirone (Buspar)
Indapamide (Lozol)	Lithium
Labetalol (Normodyne)	Some antipsychotics
Lisinopril (Zestril)	Fluphenazine (Prolixin)
Methyldopa (Aldomet)	Chlorpromazine (Thorazine)
Propranolol (Inderal)	Miscellaneous
Reserpine (Serpasil)	Carbamazepine (Tegretol)
Spironolactone (Aldactone)	Cimetidine (Tagamet) ranitidine (Zantac)
Timolol (Blocadren)	Digoxin (Lanoxin)
Antidepressants	Ethinyl estradiol (Estinyl)
Amoxapine (Asendin)	Gemfibrozil (Lopid)
Bupropion (Wellbutrin)	Hydroxyzine (Atarax)
Desipramine (Norpramin)	Ketoconazole (Nizoral)
Doxepin (Sinequan)	Medroxyprogesterone (Provera)
Fluoxetine (Prozac)	Metoclopramide (Reglan)
Imipramine (Tofranil)	Metronidazole (Flagyl)
Maprotiline (Ludiomil)	Niacin (Nicolar)
Paroxetine (Paxil)	Phentermine (Fastin)

- Referrals carry a price tag, both financially and in terms of "labeling" the patient.
- Primary care physicians have continuity with the patient and can accomplish goals during short visits.
- The patient does not feel rejected, as may occasionally happen with a referral.
- The body and mind are not falsely separated.

Where referrals are appropriate, physicians should identify a therapist in their area with expertise in marital and sexual counseling and with whom they feel comfortable. If physicians do not know of a sex therapist with whom they can consult, they can contact the Society for the Scientific Study of Sex (SSSS); the American Association for Sex Educators, Counselors, and Therapists (AASECT); or the Society for Sex Therapy and Research (SSTAR). These are professional organizations that credential sex therapists.

In a model proposed by Doherty and Baird, physicians may choose different levels of involvement with sexual issues:

Level 1. This is the baseline involvement, available to all physicians. At this level a physician addresses concerns as they are broached by the patient and provides referral to a specialist for all subsequent care.

Level 2. At this level a physician makes questioning about sexual issues a part of his or her routine care at all health maintenance visits. The physician provides education about basic anatomy, physiology, and sexual functioning, and performs a directed physical examination. If treatment requires more than simple reassurance or basic sexual education, the physician refers the patient for further care.

Level 3. At this level a physician is comfortable taking a detailed sexual history either personally or with questionnaires, performing a comprehensive physical examination, and ordering appropriate laboratory tests.

Level 4. The physician does the above and treats any organic problems that may be uncovered. Marital and/or sexual therapy is provided by a trained therapist.

Level 5. This is reserved for those family physicians who have training in marital and sexual therapy.

This model for counseling can be used by all family physicians. The PLISSIT model is another model for counseling that can be used by all family physicians:

P = *Permission.* The validation that this topic is an appropriate one to discuss with one's physician.

LI = *Limited information.* The physician provides basic medical information related to the problem.

SS = *Specific suggestions.* The physician has the knowledge to make suggestions about what things may be done to make the problem better.

IT = *Intensive therapy.* The physician undertakes the role of a therapist or refers the patient to someone else who can take on that role.

Management

Limited information is available about pharmacologic treatment of HSDD. However, the following is known. One study looking at bupropion (Wellbutrin) versus a placebo found that 63% of participants had improved symptoms. This finding was not repeated in a follow-up study. Trazodone (Desyrel), a serotonergic agent, was associated with increased libido in one study; six out of 13 depressed females reported an improvement in desire. The relationship was not related to trazedone's efficacy as an antidepressant. For women who are producing decreased levels of sex hormones, for whatever reason, testosterone has been shown in double-blind studies to profoundly affect sexual behavior. The dose used was 2.5 to 5 mg methyltestosterone (Android) Monday through Friday. Concerns regarding masculinization, adverse effects on lipids, and decreased liver function were not realized at these small physiologic doses. For patients who have prolactinemia, bromocriptine mesylate (Parlodel) 1.25 mg daily, gradually increased until the serum prolactin level is normal (usually 5 to 7.5 mg daily), improves sexual responsiveness. A host of other modalities may be useful in improving sexual functioning for a woman with HSDD (Table 8.5).

No studies have looked at how family physicians treat these sexual problems. In outcome studies of HSDD where the population under observation was patients referred to a sexual therapist, the single most important factor in positive outcomes was a spouse or partner who was motivated to work with the patient on improving the relationship. Among this same population, a combination of sexual therapy and relationship therapy most often produced the desired outcomes.

Follow-up

The frequency of follow-up visits will depend on the family physician's level of involvement. If the patient has been referred to a sexual therapist, the physician may not need to see the patient for this problem but may inquire about it at visits for other reasons. If the physician is undertaking some aspect of medical management, the

T ABLE 8.5.   Therapies that have proved useful in sexual dysfunction

Cognitive behavioral therapy	College-level sex education courses
Hypnosis	Body image workshops
Guided imagery	Massage training
Group therapy	Physical exercise classes
Communication skills training	Reading self-help books on sexual topics
Sexual attitude workshops	

Note: The choice of therapy depends on patient preference and availability of resource.

patient should be seen often enough to monitor the responsiveness to medication. If the physician has taken on a counseling role with the patient and/or her spouse, they should be seen weekly or biweekly with "homework" assignments given between visits until improvement is seen.

Patient Education

The most important thing, and perhaps the easiest, that every physician can convey to a female patient is that her body is worthy of respect and that sexuality is a natural physiologic and psychologic process.

Physicians can empower patients to learn more about their own sexuality and to take responsibility for it. This "sexual assertiveness" has been shown to lead to a higher frequency of sexual activity and orgasm, greater desire, and greater marital and sexual satisfaction.

By inquiring about inherited beliefs and values about sexuality, the physician may discover religious orthodoxy or other family-of-origin beliefs that are interfering with sexual function. This gives the physician the opportunity to help the patient "rewrite scripts."

Because relationship satisfaction plays a key role in HSDD, the physician should be prepared to offer suggestions that might promote harmony. The physician can ask the patient to keep a diary of her activities over a week, looking at how much time was spent as "family time," how much was "work time," how much was "social time," and how much was "couple time."

This simple exercise may point out how little time is being spent maintaining a healthy relationship and provides an opportunity to challenge the patient to create more time for her and her partner to be together. The physician might also encourage a couple to become involved with a marital enrichment weekend, which is offered in most areas.

DYSPAREUNIA

Dyspareunia is the experience of pain with intercourse. Women with vulvodynia comprise a subset of patients who experience pain during intercourse. Traditionally, dyspareunia has been considered a form of sexual dysfunction and, therefore, often psychologic in origin. Some, however, argue that dyspareunia is a recurrent pain syndrome, particularly when the history suggests vulvodynia.

Chief Complaints

• A 37-year-old woman mentions that she has had pain with intercourse ever since she had her second child 3 years ago.

• A 25-year-old woman presents to rule out a vaginal infection. She has noted pain with intercourse occurring right before or during her menses for the past 6 months.

Clinical Manifestations

For those who view dyspareunia primarily as a pain syndrome, patients appear to fall into a few subtypes. A carefully taken history, with emphasis on the duration of the pain, the location and quality of the pain, and the relationship to penile penetration can give guidance in determining the most likely cause.

Vulvar vestibulitis occurs most often in premenopausal women. Patients will describe pain with entry of the penis into the vagina or have pain with tampon use. Frequently, the onset of symptoms can be traced to a procedure, such as laser therapy or cryotherapy. Patients will have a positive swab test, a procedure in which a moistened cotton swab is touched to the vestibular area and the pain is reproduced. On physical examination, focal or diffuse vestibular erythema is noted.

In cyclic vulvovaginitis patients notice pain with intercourse just before or during menses. The pain may actually be worse the day following intercourse. The patient may be symptom-free on days between menses. Examination will reveal little discharge, and the amount of erythema is variable.

Essential or dysethetic vulvodynia occurs most often in perimenopausal or menopausal women. The pain is usually described as diffuse, unremitting, and burning. The degree of dyspareunia and point tenderness is less than that with vulvar vestibulitis. Physical findings are generally absent.

Other findings appearing on the physical examination that may account for pain include the following:

External genitalia
  Rigid hymen
  Painful hymenal tags
  Hymenal fibrosis
  Episiotomy scars
  Urethral caruncle
  Bartholin's cyst
  Clitoral inflammation or adhesions
  Vulvar lesions

Vagina
  Vaginal bands
  Vaginal atrophy or stenosis
  Vaginal infection
  Radiation vaginitis
  Sjögren's syndrome
  Allergic reaction to personal hygiene products

Epidemiology

The incidence of dyspareunia is not well studied. It is estimated that approximately 15% of women experience vulvar pain that interferes with sexual intercourse. The age range is the 20s to the 60s. This condition predominately affects white women. Their obstetric and gynecologic histories are otherwise unremarkable, and few have a history of sexually transmitted disease.

Risk Factors

Those who consider dyspareunia to be largely a psychosexual problem divide it into two categories: primary and secondary. It is believed that primary dyspareunia is often due to one or more of the following:

T ABLE 8.6. Most common psychosexual factors causing sexual dysfunction

Prior sexual failure	Interpersonal insecurity
Sexual performance inconsistencies	Overintellectualization at the expense of
Negative learning and attitudes about sex	sensuality
Prior sexual trauma	Sexual identity conflict
Unrealistic expectations regarding sexual performance	Sexual orientation issues
Restrictive religious beliefs	History of parent–child conflict
Sexual performance anxiety	

- Ignorance by the patient and her partner of a repertoire of lovemaking techniques that do not cause pain
- Guilt stemming from religious orthodoxy or family-of-origin beliefs that sex is shameful
- Posttraumatic stress disorder, particularly from sexual abuse
- Intrapsychic issues such as depression or anxiety

  Secondary dyspareunia is thought to stem from difficulties in the woman's current sexual relationship. Those who use this schema list several psychosexual factors that can cause dysfunction (Table 8.6).

Pathology

Histologic examination of symptomatic vestibular tissue has found the presence of chronic inflammation with infiltration of the superficial stroma. Inflammatory cells have not been found in a more widespread distribution to the glands, vessels, or nerves. Many women with pain have no pathologic findings.

Diagnosis

Table 8.7 lists medical conditions that may contribute to dyspareunia. Vaginismus is an entity to distinguish from dyspareunia. Vaginismus is marked involuntary spasm of the outer third of the vagina. The resultant pain makes penile penetration difficult. Vaginismus may occur with first sexual intercourse or first gynecologic examination, or may be acquired, in the case of sexual trauma.

T ABLE 8.7. Medical conditions that might contribute to dyspareunia

Pelvic causes	Constipation
Pelvic relaxation	Hemorrhoids
Endometriosis	Moderate to severe irritable bowel syndrome
Pelvic inflammatory disease	Urinary causes
Pelvic tumors	Cystitis
Ectopic pregnancy	Acute urethral syndrome
Gastrointestinal causes	
Proctitis	

Diagnostic Tests

When a patient describes vulvodynia, the swab test should be performed. A moistened cotton swab is gently touched to various sites along the vulva, particularly the vestibule, to see if pain is elicited. The reproduction of pain by this procedure confirms the diagnosis of vestibulitis.

Other tests to be done in the workup of vulvodynia include a microscopic examination of vaginal secretions looking for yeast and bacterial vaginosis, a urinalysis and culture, and a culture for chlamydia and gonorrhea. If the history suggests a deeper location for the pain, a pelvic ultrasound should be performed, with particular attention to the uterine adnexa and cul-de-sac. If the pain has a rectal component, anoscopy and possibly sigmoidoscopy should be done.

Referral

Many women with vulvodynia can be helped by their family physicians. Patients with refractory symptoms that do not improve with conservative treatment may benefit from referral to a gynecologist with expertise in this area for further evaluation and consideration of possible surgical therapy. Women whose dyspareunia appears to stem from more deep-seated psychosexual issues may benefit from referral to a couple's therapist with expertise in sex therapy.

Management

Table 8.8 lists the treatments that have been shown to be helpful for vulvodynia.

Follow-up

For a family physician who is actively involved in the care of a patient with vulvodynia, visits should be scheduled at monthly intervals, at least initially, to monitor for improvement in pain and in the patient's sexual relationship. If improvement seems persistent, the problem can be addressed at the patient's yearly visit. If no progress is apparent or if the pain improves but the patient and her partner continue to have difficulties with their sexual relationship, referral to a sex therapist should be considered.

T **ABLE 8.8.** Treatments found to be helpful in vulvodynia

Vulvar vestibulitis	Topical estradiol cream,* 0.01% twice daily
	Intralesional interferon injection
	Physical therapy with biofeedback
	Low-oxalate diet
	Oral calcium citrate*
	Support groups
Cyclic vulvovaginitis	Empiric trial with fluconazole (Diflucan),* 150 mg weekly for 2 months, then twice monthly for 2 to 4 months; monitor liver function
	Physical therapy with biofeedback
	Low-oxalate diet
	Oral calcium citrate*
	Support groups
Essential or dysesthetic vulvodynia	Tricyclic antidepressants* in gradually increasing doses for up to 6 months
	Physical therapy with biofeedback
	Support groups

*Not approved for this use by the U.S. Food and Drug Administration.

Patient Education

Patients should be commended for their willingness to deal with this sensitive and difficult issue. The physician may again take this opportunity to emphasize that sexuality is normal and healthy. Those whose sexual lives are not satisfying should be validated in their attempts to work with their physicians and other professionals to make them more satisfactory.

ORGASMIC DISORDERS

Female orgasmic disorder is defined as a persistent or recurrent delay in or absence of orgasm following a normal sexual excitement phase. This condition can cause distress or marked interpersonal difficulty.

Chief Complaint

- A 25-year-old woman comes in for a Pap smear. She has never been married and has not been involved in many relationships. When you ask about sexual difficulties, she mentions that she has never experienced orgasm. For this reason she has avoided intimate relationships and worries that marriage and motherhood are not possible for her.

Clinical Manifestations

This *Diagnostic and Statistical Manual IV* (DSM-IV) diagnosis may be present in all sexual situations or may occur only in certain settings. Once a woman has learned how to achieve orgasm, it is unusual for her to lose that ability (Table 8.9).

T ABLE 8.9. Diagnostic criteria for 302.73 female orgasmic disorder

A. Persistent or recurrent delay in, or absence of, orgasm following a normal sexual excitement phase. Women exhibit wide variability in the type or intensity of stimulation that triggers orgasm. The diagnosis of female orgasmic disorder should be based on the clinician's judgment that the woman's orgasmic capability is less than would be reasonable for her age, sexual experience, and the adequacy of sexual stimulation she receives.

B. The disturbance causes marked distress or interpersonal difficulty.

C. The orgasmic dysfunction is not better accounted for by another Axis I disorder (except another sexual dysfunction) and is not due exclusively to the direct physiological effects of a substance (e.g., a drug of abuse, a medication) or a general medical condition.

Specify type:

        Lifelong type
        Acquired type

Specify type:

        Generalized type
        Situational type

Specify:

        Due to psychological factors
        Due to combined factors

Reprinted with permission from *Diagnostic and Statistical Manual of Mental Disorders,* 4th ed. rev. Washington, D.C.: American Psychiatric Association, 1995.

Epidemiology

One study of couples recruited through community groups found that 46% of the female respondents reported difficulty reaching orgasm, and 15% said they were anorgasmic. Couples were enrolled in the study if they reported their marriage was working well.

Risk Factors

The following experiences can cause orgasmic difficulty in women who were previously orgasmic:

• Poor sexual communication
• Relationship conflict
• A traumatic experience, particularly sexual assault
• A mood disorder
• General medical disorders
    Several common pharmacologic agents are known to inhibit orgasm (Table 8.10).

Pathology

Other than pharmacologic causes, there are no known organic causes of primary anorgasmia.

Diagnosis

As with the other sexual dysfunctions covered in this chapter, orgasmic disorders can be uncovered by a detailed sexual history with questions about orgasmic response.

Referral

Again, the decision to treat or refer rests partly in the family physician's comfort with undertaking treatment. Physicians who are not interested in attempting treatment may refer patients as soon as the problem is discovered. Other physicians who choose to undertake treatment may wish to consider referral to a sex therapist if there is no progress after several visits with the patient.

Management

One technique in the treatment of orgasmic disorder proceeds in a sequence of steps:

TABLE 8.10. Commonly used agents that have been reported to cause orgasmic difficulties

Amoxapine (Asendin)
Benzodiazepines
Clonidine (Catapres)
Fluoxetine (Prozac)
Imipramine (Tofranil)
Nortriptyline (Pamelor)
Paroxetine (Paxil)
Phentermine (Fastin)
Sertraline (Zoloft)
Trazodone (Desyrel)
Venlafaxine (Effexor)

1. The first step is an assessment of sexual attitudes, particularly those regarding the importance of orgasm.
2. The patient then is educated about basic anatomy and physiology, with an emphasis on those parts of the female anatomy that respond most to stimulation. The use of drawings or models is helpful here, but perhaps even more useful is the so-called educational pelvic examination in which a woman is shown her own anatomy by means of a hand-held mirror.
3. The woman is then encouraged to explore her body visually and with touch. This can be assigned as homework or can be an exercise done, with informed consent, first by her physician and then by herself in the presence of her partner. The physician can apply light touch, starting posteriorly at the introitus and then moving laterally and anteriorly, while the woman notes where touch feels most pleasurable.
4. The woman is then asked to stimulate herself at home manually or with a vibrator until she experiences orgasm.
5. Once she has achieved orgasm, she should be instructed to develop fantasies that accompany the orgasmic experience.
6. To avoid undue focus on orgasm as the only acceptable outcome of sexual activity, the woman should be encouraged to then practice sensate focusing, a technique originated by Masters and Johnson. This technique involves carving out undisturbed time to focus on those bodily sensations that are pleasurable. Pleasurable sensations may be not only tactile but olfactory, visual, and auditory. The woman may explore all of her body, not just her genital area.
7. At first the sensate focusing is done by the patient alone; then, after comfort has been achieved, it is done in conjunction with her partner.

Couples should be told to experiment with different positions during intercourse that provide more constant contact between the penis and the clitoris. The use of Kegel exercises has also been found to be useful in women who have difficulty achieving orgasm. Conditioning the perivaginal muscles increases female arousal and facilitates orgasm. Part of the "educational pelvic examination" might include having the woman tighten her vaginal muscles around the examiner's fingers to identify the muscles involved in Kegel exercises.

Follow-up

The process outlined previously is a multistep one that takes place over a series of weeks, with the patient given homework to do between sessions. She should be seen frequently enough to be supported in this endeavor. When orgasm has been achieved as part of her sexual relationship, follow-up can occur at her yearly examination or as needed.

Patient Education

As with the other sexual dysfunctions, the greatest service a physician can provide is normalization of sexual activity and permission to seek a satisfying relationship. Patients can be helped to be more assertive about making their wishes known to their sexual partners.

SUGGESTED READINGS

Beck JG. Hypoactive sexual desire disorder: an overview. *J Consult Clin Psych* 1995: 63:919.

Butcher J. Female sexual problems: Loss of desire—what about the fun? *Br Med J* 1999;318:41.

Doherty WJ, Baird MA. Developmental levels in family-centered medical care. *Fam Med* 1986;18:153–156.

Finger WW, Lund M, Slagle MA. Medications that may contribute to sexual disorders. *J Fam Prac* 1997; 44:33.

Halvorsen JG, Metz ME. Sexual dysfunction, part I: Classification, etiology and pathogenesis. *J Am Board Fam Prac* 1992;5:51.

Halvorsen JG, Metz ME. Sexual dysfunction, part II: Diagnosis, management, and prognosis. *J Am Board Fam Prac* 1992;5:177.

Laumann EO, Paik A, Rosen R. Sexual dysfunction in the United Satets: Prevalence and predictors. *JAMA* 1999;281:537.

Meana M, Binik YM, Khalife S, Cohen D. Dyspareunia: Sexual dysfunction or pain syndrome? *J Nerv Men Dis* 1997;185:561.

Metts JF. Vulvodynia and vulvar vestibulitis: Challenges in diagnosis and management. *Am Fam Physician* 1999;59:1547.

Pagano R. Vulvar vestibulitis syndrome:an often unrecognized cause of dyspareunia. *Australia N Z J Obs Gynaecol* 1999; 39:79.

Rosen RC, Leiblum SR. Hypoactive sexual desire. *Psych Cl North Am* 1995;18(1):107.

Stuart M, Lieberman J. *The fifteen minute hour: applied psychotherapy for the primary care physician,* 2nd ed. Westport, CT: Praeger, 1993.

Warnock JK, Bundren JC, Morris DW. Female hypoactive sexual desire disorder due to androgen deficiency: Clinical and psychometric issues. *Psychopharm Bull* 1997; 33:761.

CHAPTER 9

Osteoarthritis, Rheumatoid Arthritis, and Osteoporosis

Jo Ann Rosenfeld

Osteoarthritis, rheumatoid arthritis, and osteoporosis cause significant pain, disability, loss of independence, and cost to the elderly. All three diseases occur more commonly in women.

OSTEOARTHRITIS

Osteoarthritis (OA) is a common cause of physical impairment in the elderly. It is a degenerative disease of the cartilage of joints that occurs as a result of both mechanical and biologic events. It has multiple etiologies and a slowly progressive course.

Chief Complaint
- A 64-year-old woman presents with knee pain, swelling, joint pain, and stiffness. The pain is usually worse late in the day. Morning stiffness usually lasts less than 30 minutes.

Clinical Manifestations
OA usually affects single large joints such as the knee and hip and/or the first or distal interphalangeal (DIP) joints (causing Heberden's nodes) and proximal interphalangeal joints, and the base of the thumb. Metacarpal, metacarpophalangeal joints, wrists, and ankles are usually spared. The disease has a waxing and waning course, and its rate of progression varies.

Epidemiology
- OA is the most common cause of arthritis, accounting for three out of four cases of symptomatic arthritis.
- It is projected that by 2020 in the United States, 59 million older adults will have some arthritis.
- OA of the knee is the most common joint disorder. Radiographic changes of the knee are present in one-third of individuals greater than 65 years of age.

Risk Factors
   Risk factors are summarized in Fig. 9.1.
- **Sex.** According to prospective long-term population studies, being a woman is a risk factor for OA. Women are twice as likely to develop OA as men.
- **Age.** The incidence of OA increases more rapidly with age in women, particularly OA of the small joints of the hand. Women have a plateau in incidence after age 60,

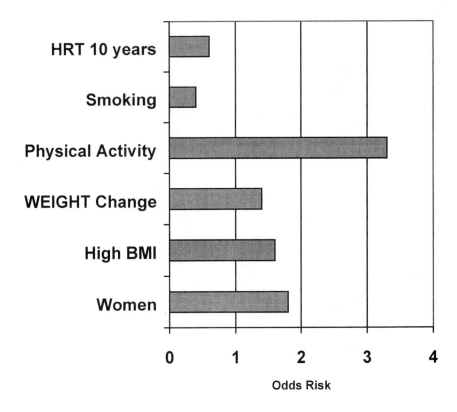

FIGURE 9.1. Risk factors for osteoarthritis. HRT, hormone replacement therapy; BMI, body mass index.

compared with men, who have a slower rise that continues into the seventh and eighth decades.

- **Excessive weight.** A high baseline body mass index (BMI) or a rapid weight gain increases the risk of OA. The risk of developing OA increases with each 10-pound weight increase.
- **Physical activity.** This appears to increase the risk of OA. However, long-term, long-distance runners had a significantly lower degree of disability and mortality. This effect was much more significant for women than for men.
- **Decreased risk.** Several factors have been linked with a decreased risk of OA. These include smoking and using hormone replacement therapy (HRT). The effect of HRT on OA is controversial. In some studies there is an inverse association between HRT and risk of OA; in others the relative risk for OA in women who use HRT is 1.0. HRT is associated with a lower than expected risk of knee and hip arthritis.

Diagnosis

OA is a clinical diagnosis based on joint pain, joint stiffness of less than 30 minutes in the morning, and lack of systemic symptoms. The pain is usually poorly localized, asymmetric, and episodic. At first, pain occurs with activity, but as the disease progresses, the pain also occurs at rest.

The American College of Rheumatology has established the following classification criteria for OA of the hip. Hip pain and at least two of the following three items:
- Erythrocyte sedimentation rate (ESR) of less than 20 mm/hr
- Radiographic femoral or acetabular osteophytes
- Radiographic joint pain narrowing

The American College of Rheumatology has established the following classification criteria for OA of the knee. Knee pain and radiographic osteophytes and at least one of the following three items:
- Age less than 50 years
- Morning stiffness of less than 30 minutes each morning
- Crepitus on motion
- **Physical examination.** The large joints often do not show heat or redness. Affected joints are often tender on pressure, are swollen, and show crepitus with movement. There may be joint line tenderness. Late in the disease, the patient may show signs of decreased muscle strength, reduced range of motion, and contractures.
- **Radiographs.** Radiographic findings do not correlate with severity of pain or disability; they do correlate with the severity of joint pathology. Findings include osteophytes, joint space narrowing, and subchondral sclerosis.
- **Diagnostic aspiration of inflamed joint.** The fluid should be sent for white blood count (WBC) and differential, crystal analysis, Gram's stain, and culture. The WBC is high in inflammation, and even higher in infection. If infection is suspected, radiographs of joints and complete blood count (CBC) and blood cultures are appropriate. Infection and crystalline arthritis can occur in the same joint, because infection is more likely in a damaged joint.

The differential diagnosis can be found in Table 9.1.

Management

The goals of treatment are to reduce pain, maintain function, minimize disability, educate the patient, protect the joint, and prevent iatrogenic injury. Medical treatment must be individualized and often includes many of the following:
- Stabilization of coexisting disease
- Social and psychologic support

T ABLE 9.1. Differential diagnosis of osteoarthritis

Crystalline arthritis
  Calcium pyrophosphate disease
  Gout
Connective tissue arthritides
  Rheumatoid arthritis
  Psoriatic arthritis
Infective arthritides
  Septic arthritis
  Lyme arthritis
Traumatic arthritis

- Physiotherapy and occupational therapy
- Exercise, active or passive, to keep up muscular conditioning, improve strength, and maintain function
- Reduction in body weight
- Use of assistive devices—canes, walkers, braces
- Self-management programs
- Pain control

Pain control should be started with acetaminophen. Up to 1,000 mg four times a day is the preferred first-line therapy. Nonsteroidal anti-inflammatory drugs (NSAIDs) should be avoided if possible. If used, low doses of NSAIDs should be given for pain control, rather than the customary anti-inflammatory doses.

NSAIDs can have severe side effects (Table 9.2), especially in the elderly, including upper gastrointestinal bleeding. Gastric ulcers occur in 15% of the elderly who chronically use NSAIDs. Edema, hyponatremia, hyperkalemia, and renal and hepatic toxicity can also occur. Some experts suggest that NSAIDs may affect normal cartilage and accelerate breakdown of articular cartilage.

There is no place for systemic steroids or narcotics in the treatment of OA. Intraarticular steroid injection can be given in a single joint. This is warranted with single swollen or tender joints. However, it should be used infrequently.

Referral

Surgery is indicated in some patients with severe disease. Joint replacement or arthroscopy with debridement of cartilage and washout of joint space may be helpful. The risks of surgery have decreased with new technologies, including prosthetic devices and new surgical techniques. Total hip replacement is an option for patients with disease of the hip and the following:

- Chronic discomfort
- Considerable impairment
- Joint failure caused by OA, rheumatoid arthritis, avascular necrosis, traumatic arthritis, hip fractures, bone turners, Paget's disease arthritis, ankylosing spondylitis, and/or juvenile rheumatoid arthritis
- Radiographic evidence of joint damage
- Moderate to severe persistent pain, severe disability, or both, not relieved by an extended course of nonsurgical management

The goals of hip replacement include relief of pain and improvement of function.

Follow-up

Women with OA need close follow-up every 1 to 3 months, depending on the severity of the disease. Examine joint mobility and ask about activities of daily living and how arthritis affects them.

T ABLE 9.2.   **Risk factors for gastrointestinal or renal complications of NSAIDs**

Age more than 65 years
History of peptic ulcer disease or upper gastrointestinal bleeding
Hypertension
Congestive heart failure
Use of steroids, anticoagulants, diuretics, or angiotensin-converting enzyme (ACE) inhibitors
Tobacco use
Alcohol use

Abbreviation: NSAIDs, nonsteroidal anti-inflammatory drugs.

RHEUMATOID ARTHRITIS

Rheumatoid arthritis (RA) is a systemic inflammatory connective-tissue disease in which a destructive arthritis is often a predominant feature. Systemic symptoms of fatigue, anemia, weight loss, fever, and malaise often occur. RA is progressive and destructive, and causes significant disability and distortion.

Chief Complaints
- A 32-year-old woman with sudden onset of bilateral hand and wrist swelling
- A 44-year-old woman with an acutely swollen hot red knee
- A 64-year-old woman with fatigue, weight loss, myalgia, hip pain, and a vascular rash on the pretibial surfaces of her legs

CLINICAL MANIFESTATIONS
RA is a connective-tissue disease that can involve any synovial-lined joint. The most frequently involved joints are the small joints of the hands and feet, wrists, knees, and elbows, and the gelenohumeral and acromioclavicular joints. Most women commonly show bilateral symmetric disease, although it can present asymmetrically, especially when one joint is used more than others. RA occurs in two forms: acute single or multiple joint arthritis, or an insidious form with multiple systemic manifestations, including pericarditis and pleuritis. The arthritis can vary from a mild form to one that is crippling, disabling, and destructive. Systemic symptoms can precede the arthritis and include anorexia, malaise, fatigue, weight loss, fever, myalgia, sweats, and paresthesias. The disease often waxes and wanes over weeks to years, with remissions and exacerbations occurring spontaneously. The symptoms of RA are generally less severe in the second half of the menstrual cycle and during pregnancy. The disease rebounds in intensity postpartum.

Epidemiology
- Among the general population, 0.4% has RA.
- RA can occur at any age, but its peak occurrence is in 30- to 50-year-olds.
- Women have an increased incidence, with a ratio of 3:1 when compared with men.

Risk Factors
Risk factors for women include increased parity and breastfeeding. Women who have more than three children have an increased risk of developing severe RA (relative risk = 4.8), and an increased risk of poor prognosis. Forty-six percent of women with severe RA had a history of breastfeeding more than 6 months, as compared with 26% of controls.

A history of oral contraceptive pill (OCP) use is associated with a decreased risk of RA. Using OCPs for more than 5 years decreased the relative risk of developing severe disease to 0.1 after correcting for age, parity, and breastfeeding.

Magnetic resonance imaging (MRI) is the next best diagnostic test after radiographs. MRI is indicated when diagnosis is uncertain.

Pathology
The pathology is acute and chronic inflammation of chondral joints and systemic signs of inflammation.

Diagnosis
The diagnosis is clinical and usually documented over a period of months to years. Early in the disease, the radiographic findings may not be symmetric, but with time they may become so. The appendicular skeleton is more involved than the apical skeleton. Often there are osseous and soft-tissue manifestations. Findings include

fusiform and periarticular soft-tissue swelling, juxtaarticular osteoporosis, uniform joint space loss, and marginal erosions.

In larger joints, radiographic findings include narrowing of the joint space and osteoporosis. The hip may show axial migration into the pelvis, and the shoulder may show rotator cuff injury and subacromial bursitis.

Patients with RA usually have a normochromic normocytic anemia, although it can be microcytic. The ESR and C-reactive protein are usually elevated. Rheumatoid factor (RF) is present in more than 60% of those with the disease, but it is also present in 5% of normal individuals. Joint fluid analysis shows a high white blood count, with normal glucose and increased protein.

Referral

All women with RA need early referral to physicians comfortable in using disease-modifying drugs such as methotrexate (Rheumatrox) and hydroxychloroquine sulfate (Plaquenil) to preserve joint function and improve prognosis. Surgeons may be needed for joint replacement when pain or disability is significant.

Management

Treatment includes pain management, anti-inflammatory drugs, and drugs to reduce the destruction of the joint. Use of HRT does not improve the course or prognosis of women with RA. However, one small randomized control trial showed that testosterone given to women with RA produced a significant improvement.

OSTEOPOROSIS

Osteoporosis (OP) is a condition in which an individual has low bone mass. This results in an increased risk of fracture.

Chief Complaints
- A 45-year-old woman with Colles' fracture of the right wrist
- A 54-year-old menopausal woman contemplating HRT
- A 74-year-old woman with pain from vertebral fractures and kyphoscoliosis

Epidemiology
- One in six white women will have a hip fracture in her lifetime.
- Fifty-four percent of women who are currently 50 years of age will have an OP-related fracture during their lifetimes.
- Spinal fractures caused by OP occur in 25% of white women by age 65. These fractures carry a mortality rate of 5% to 20% within the first year after fracture. Ten percent of women with a hip fracture become dependent.

Risk Factors
Risk factors for OP include the following (Table 9.3):
- White and Asian races
- Lower body weight or losing weight. Woman who lose weight over 2 years are more likely to have increased risk of subsequent nonspine fractures
- Cigarette smoking
- Menopause
- Sedentary lifestyle
- Family history
- Nutrition (low calcium)
- Alcoholism
- Early menopause

TABLE 9.3. **Risk factors for osteoporosis**

Diet/lifestyle
    Low lifelong calcium intake
    High salt intake
    Smoking
    High caffeine intake
    High protein intake
    Excessive alcohol intake
    Lack of exercise
History
    White or Asian ethnicity
    Thin body habitus
    Family history of osteoporosis
Female factors
    Early menopause
    Nulliparity
    Early surgical menopause
Medical factors
    Hyperthyroidism

Risk factors for hip fractures from OP (Table 9.4) include the following:
- Loss of weight
- Tallness
- High caffeine intake

Other diseases and medication use are associated with OP. Use of corticosteroids, antiseizure medications, and some chemotherapeutic agents may increase the risk of

TABLE 9.4. **Risk factors for hip fracture in women**

Losing weight
Tallness
High caffeine intake
Older age
History of maternal hip fracture
Poor self-rated health
Previous hyperthyroidism
Current use of long-acting benzodiazepines
Current use of anticonvulsant drugs
Being on feet less than 4 hours a day
Low distant depth perception
Resting pulse >80 beats per minute
Any fracture after age 50

OP. Several factors are not associated with increased risk of hip fracture, including ethnicity, number of children, history of breastfeeding, timing of menopause, past smoking status, use of short-acting benzodiazepines, and levels of dietary calcium.

Smoking was not a risk factor when controlled for weight and health.

Prevention

Primary prevention of hip and other fractures includes routine assessment of all elderly women for risk of OP, including the following:
- Use of HRT
- Diet
- Physical activity
- Consideration of other medical conditions

Use of HRT in postmenopausal women is both preventive and protective. HRT is the cornerstone of preventive therapy for OP and fractures (Fig. 9.2). Current users of estrogen have decreased risk for hip, wrist, and spine fractures. Estrogen use and exercise actually increased bone density values in women with low bone density after 2 years. Concomitant use of progesterone does not decrease the benefit of estrogen use on OP prevention or treatment.

However, it is unclear when HRT should be started and how long it must be used for optimal prevention and treatment of OP. The risk of OP is decreased the greatest among current or recent users of HRT. The decrease in risk diminishes with time after stopping estrogen. Whether a history of HRT use confers benefits is unclear.

The magnitude of HRT effect on OP was greater if it was started earlier in menopause, and the effect was diminished if HRT was initiated more than 5 years after menopause. Being over the age of 75 or a smoker does not decrease the benefit of estrogen. The minimally effective daily dosage of estrogen is 0.625 mg oral conju-

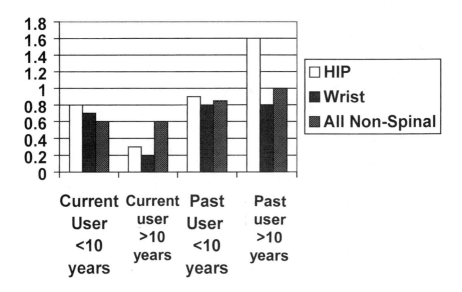

FIGURE 9.2. The relative risk of fracture for women with HRT use.

gated equine estrogen, 1.0 mg oral estradiol, or 50 to 100 mg of transdermal estradiol per day. Premenopausal women who develop amenorrhea related to anorexia, low body weight, or excessive exercise are also at risk for OP, and their bone mass may be protected by using OCPs. Low-dose OCPs offer protection from the development of osteoporosis. Whether premenopausal women who use long-term depo-medroxy-progesterone (Depo-Provera) or implantable progesterone (Norplant) are at increased risk for OP is unclear.

Other preventive methods include the use of calcium and vitamin D. Post-menopausal women need 1,000 to 1,500 mg elemental calcium daily (4- to 8-ounce glasses of milk). The main side effect is constipation. In elderly women, as little as 1,000 mg of calcium daily may retard bone loss.

Diagnosis

Some **laboratory tests** may help to evaluate the woman suspected of having OP. Calcium levels and alkaline phosphate levels are normal in OP but abnormal in metabolic bone diseases such as hyperparathyroidism and vitamin D deficiency–induced osteopenia. Thyroid-stimulating hormone (TSH) levels should be determined in women with hypothyroidism. Women receiving thyroid replacement who have low TSH levels may have excessive bone loss. Thyroid hormone replacement should be reduced. Bone pain or a history of fractures would be consistent with OP. On physical examination, kyphoscoliosis or signs of fractures would suggest OP. Other tests may be needed to exclude other causes of osteopenia; a serum protein electrophoresis may be needed if multiple myeloma is suggested. Bone protein metabolite assays of blood and urine for breakdown products of bone to determine the presence and degree of bone loss are controversial. These measure bone-specific alkaline phosphotase or collagen products, but the relationship of these levels to OP and risk of fracture is unclear.

Standard radiographs do not determine early or mild loss. Bone mineral densitometry is useful. Medicare now pays for a screening bone densitometry reading every 2 years. Treatment is recommended when values are two or more standard deviations below peak bone mass (not corrected for age). Absorptiometry of lumbar spine and hip provides the most precise measure.

Management

Treatment must be individualized, considering risk factors for use of HRT and comorbid conditions.

Recommendations of the National Institutes of Health (NIH) Conference on Management of Osteoporosis include the following:
• Estrogen therapy
• Calcium supplementation started at age 40, or at approximately 10 years before menopause (1,000 mg elemental calcium daily)
• Weight-bearing exercise (e.g., walking, jogging, rowing, weight lifting)

Other Treatments

Biphosphonates are synthetic pyrophosphate analogs that prevent bone resorption through inhibition of osteoclastic activity. Etidronate (Didronel) inhibits bone formation and prevents bone resorption (it is not approved by the FDA for use in OP), but a more recently released product, alendronate (Fosamax) (10 mg daily), does not inhibit bone formation. However, it is more expensive than etidronate.

Alendronate results in a bone mineral density increase of 8.8% in the spine and 6.9% in the femoral neck with 2 years' use. The incidence of vertebral compression fractures was reduced by 48% with use. Side effects include gastrointestinal (GI) symptoms of pain, nausea, constipation, and diarrhea. It must be taken with 8 ounces of water on awakening, at least one half-hour before food, drink, and medication.

Calcitonin deficiency has not been proved to cause OP. Nonetheless, treatment with exogenous calcitonin has an antiresportive effect, albeit a short-term one (only 1 to 2 years).

The usual dosage is 100 IU salmon preparation or 0.5 mg of recombinant form subcutaneously (Calcimar) three times per week. Bedtime injections may decrease facial flushing and nausea. Intranasal salmon calcitonin (Miacalcin) is available but has not been approved by all pharmacy plants. The daily dosage is 200 IU in alternating nostrils. This causes no nausea but does cause local nasal irritation.

Research suggests that **fluoride** stimulates osteoblast function, but it may increase the fracture incidence. (The FDA has not approved fluoride for this use.) The dosage is 45 to 75 mg daily. In addition, fluoride has GI side effects.

Research has also suggested that intermittent low-dose **parathyroid hormone** stimulates bone formation, whereas high doses cause bone resorption. However, its use for treatment is not yet advised.

In small trials, use of growth hormone releasing hormone (GHRH) and growth hormone (GH) has increased lumbar bone density.

Follow-up

After an initial bone densitometry reading showing OP, and initiation of therapy, 2 years of therapy are necessary before repeat densitometry can be used to evaluate for effectiveness of treatment. Treatment of OP is a multiyear commitment.

CHAPTER 10

Fibromyalgia and Chronic Fatigue Syndrome

C. Carolyn Thiedke

FIBROMYALGIA

Fibromyalgia and chronic fatigue syndrome present real challenges for physicians. The degree of patients' suffering and disability, the lack of major physical or laboratory findings, the elusiveness of known pathogenesis, and the paucity of effective treatment options combine to frustrate physicians. Unfortunately, physicians have often communicated their frustrations to patients.

Patients, in turn, become frustrated, and many travel from doctor to doctor hoping to find one who will listen to their complaints sympathetically and work with them to improve their lives. Family physicians, with their generalist training and their comfort with working with patients over time, are well qualified to provide care for these patients.

Definition

Fibromyalgia (FM) is a common clinical condition whose hallmark, and chief reproducible finding, is the presence of multiple tender points. This finding is commonly accompanied by generalized body ache, morning stiffness, fatigue, and nonrestful sleep.

A significant majority of patients troubled by fibromyalgia are women. As a group, patients with FM visit their physicians more than patients with other chronic illnesses. Thus it is likely that patients with FM will represent a significant proportion of the women most often seen by a family physician.

Chief Complaint

- A 43-year-old female accountant and mother of two comes in because she hurts all over. She feels exhausted much of the time. She has read about fibromyalgia and wonders if this might be what is affecting her.

Clinical Manifestations

Although the clinical picture that we call fibromyalgia today was described as far back as the nineteenth century, the American College of Rheumatology issued consensus criteria as recently as 1990. The sine qua non is the finding of nine pairs of tender points, scattered over the torso and extremities. The patient must report pain on digital pressure in at least 11 of these 18 potential tender-point sites (Fig. 10.1). These tender points have been studied and validated, and their presence has been found to have acceptable degrees of sensitivity and specificity for this diagnosis.

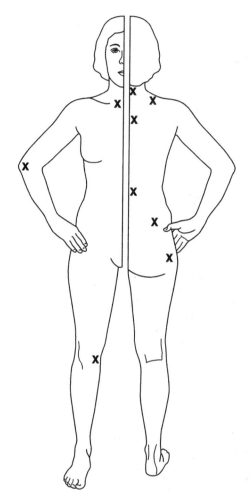

FIGURE 10.1. Location of tender points in fibromyalgia—the nine pairs of tender points used for the American College of Rheumatology diagnostic criteria study of fibromyalgia. Each site should be tender bilaterally on digital palpation.

Additionally, the following diagnostic points have been found to help confirm the diagnosis of FM:
- Diffuse muscle aching
- Pain complaints that include radiation from the torso over large areas of the body; bilateral, above and below the waist, and along the axial skeleton; no diurnal variation but variation with the weather

Other musculoskeletal complaints include morning stiffness (lasting less than 1 hour on arising), joint swelling (although none is demonstrable), hypermobility, and carpal tunnel-like symptoms.

Noted almost as frequently as pain is nonrestful sleep. Indeed, Moldofsky and associates demonstrated an anomalous sleep electroencephalography (EEG) pattern in patients with FM. When this alpha non-REM (NREM) pattern was induced in healthy volunteers with normal sleep, they demonstrated increased tenderness as well.

Other, less commonly associated conditions include the following:
- Irritable bowel syndrome
- Raynaud's phenomenon
- Headache
- Nondermatomal paresthesia
- Psychic distress
- Marked functional impairment (the unemployment rate among patients with FM is 36%.)

Epidemiology

FM is a syndrome that occurs predominantly in young and middle-aged females. It is a phenomenon generally seen in the upper and middle classes. Although the populations initially studied contained predominantly white women, FM is now being noted among other ethnic groups as well.

Population studies have put the prevalence anywhere from 0.7% to 13% of adult women. Studies done in primary care populations suggest a prevalence of 1.9% to 3.7% (men and women).

Family studies of patients with FM have found high rates of depression and other affective disorders among family members.

Risk Factors

FM, particularly when first receiving wider recognition, was generally attributed to a physical stressor. A virus was the most frequently accepted cause because many patients link the onset of illness with a flulike prodrome. Trauma appeared to be an inciting factor in others.

As time has passed other causes have been postulated:
- A primary psychiatric disturbance
- A sleep disturbance
- Prolonged inactivity leading to deconditioning

A more apt description may be to say it is a **stress-related illness** because the onset frequently coincides with a period of increased emotional or physical stress and the severity of symptoms is strongly influenced by a patient's perceived level of stress.

It appears that when a significant stressor occurs in someone who is predisposed, perhaps genetically, the response is a high degree of anxiety, which in turn leads to a maladaptive behavior response. The response may include the following:
- Decreased level of function
- Increased sensitivity to pain
- Inactivity

All these findings could stem from central nervous system (CNS) changes that cause the following:
- Disordered Stage 4 sleep
- Upregulation of the sympathetic nervous system, leading to changes in muscle perfusion and pain thresholds
- Changes in the functional activity of the caudate nucleus and thalamus

When compared with patients who have rheumatoid arthritis and normal controls, FM patients report more distress, especially life stress and "daily hassles." There is a direct correlation between the degree of psychic distress and the number of tender points.

Some researchers who have studied FM believe that it and major depressive disorders are part of a wider spectrum of related disorders. Others note that the populations who have generally been studied are those that present to rheumatologists and are a "sicker" group, and that studies of FM in the general population reveal no greater psychiatric comorbidity.

Pathology

Because the cause of FM has been elusive, numerous hypotheses have been promoted. FM has been proposed to be caused by the following:

- Hypothalamic dysfunction
- Limbic system dysfunction
- Chronobiologic disturbance
- Serotonin deficit
- General disturbance in the modulation of nervous system tone
    Some of the findings that support these hypotheses are the following:
- Abnormal alpha sleep EEG patterns
- Lower urinary free cortisol levels
- Low blood levels of serotonin
- Low cerebrospinal (CSF) levels of serotonin
- Lower levels of circulating somatomedin C
- Higher levels of substance P in the CSF

Two research groups have reported that patients with FM have lower than normal levels of natural killer T-cell activity. Others have reported a decrease in the number of T cells expressing activation markers and a change in interleukin-2 secretion by activated T cells. The significance of these findings is unknown. Currently, there is no evidence that FM is related to a specific defect in the immune system or to a particular infectious disease (despite the finding that 55% of patients recall a flulike illness at the start of their FM).

Although the hallmark of FM is muscle pain, examination of muscle tissue via microscope, electron microscope, electromyography, muscle metabolism studies, and nuclear magnetic resonance (MR) spectroscopy has failed to reveal any difference between the muscle tissue of FM patients and that of controls.

Recent research looking at central processing of pain suggests that insults to the brain can forever change the way that pain is perceived. Thus FM may not be a peripheral problem at all, but rather a central one. Studies using single photon emission computed tomographic (SPECT) scans support that. Researchers have found decreased regional blood flow to the thalamus and caudate nucleus in patients with FM. These are the centers of the brain that deal with pain perception. SPECT studies in patients with neuropathic pain and metastatic cancer show similar patterns.

Diagnosis

The differential diagnosis of FM is listed in Table 10.1. Tender points found with FM should be distinguished from "trigger points." Trigger points do not radiate, there is no pain distal to the examiner's finger, and they are not generally bilateral. Trigger points are more often single. Trigger points are found sporadically in the general population and are not associated with an underlying condition. They are most likely related to an overuse injury.

Although a thorough history and careful physical examination are the best tools to distinguish FM from other diseases, the initial evaluation should include a complete blood count (CBC), sedimentation rate, fasting blood sugar, and evaluation of thyroid-stimulating hormone (TSH) levels.

Unless patients have symptoms suggestive of narcolepsy (e.g., falling asleep at the wheel of a car or inability to stay awake during situations that require arousal), a sleep study is not indicated.

When considering the diagnosis of FM, physicians should screen for diagnosable psychiatric illness, particularly depression and anxiety, using a screening questionnaire or a structured diagnostic interview.

T ABLE 10.1. Differential diagnosis of fibromyalgia

Idiopathic
    Polymyositis/dermatomyositis complex
    Inclusion body myositis
Infectious myositis
    Bacterial
    Viral
    Fungal
    Parasitic
Drug-induced myopathic syndrome
Endocrinopathies
    Hypothyroidism
    Hyperthyroidism
Myositis associated with collagen vascular disease
Polymyalgia rheumatica and temporal arteritis
Occult or metastatic cancer
Neuromuscular disease
    Myasthenia gravis
    Amyotrophic lateral sclerosis
    Familial periodic paralysis
Guillain-Barré syndrome
Diabetes mellitus
Porphyria

Referral

Most patients with FM can be managed by the family physician with whom they have a long-term relationship. However, physicians may wish to seek out and cultivate relationships in their communities with those who have expertise in exercise therapy, biofeedback, hypnotherapy, yoga, tai chi, and cognitive behavior therapy.

Management

The predominant medications that have been found to be helpful in FM are the tricyclic antidepressants (TCAs), particularly amitriptyline (Elavil). They appear to help the patient to

- Decrease pain at tender points
- Improve sleep quality
- Decrease fatigue
- Decrease morning stiffness
- Improve depression
- Improve anxiety

    Doses of from 10 to 100 mg of amitriptyline at bedtime are usually effective and have minimal side effects. Cyclobenzaprine (Flexeril), 10 mg at bedtime, has also been found to be helpful. The serotonin reuptake inhibitors (SSRIs) have not been found to be particularly helpful in FM, although they are worth a try if the patient has no response to TCAs. One study showed that a combination of fluoxetine (Prozac) and amitriptyline was superior to either alone. Another found that a combination of alprazolam (Xanax) and ibuprofen (Motrin) decreased the number of tender points and the patient's assessment of the severity of symptoms. Nonsteroidal anti-inflammatory drugs (NSAIDs) such as ibuprofen and naproxen (Naprosyn) have not shown significant benefit for FM.

S-adenosyl-L-methionine (SAM-e) is a naturally occurring active derivative of methionine that is present in all body tissue. In several studies, SAM was found to be superior to placebo in producing improvement of symptoms. It is currently available as an over-the-counter supplement in the United States.

Some patients with FM may have a sleep disorder, predominantly periodic limb movement or nocturnal myoclonus. This can be treated with carbidopa/levodopa (Sinemet) 10/100 or clonazepam (Klonopin) 0.5 mg with the evening meal.

If a patient with FM appears to have a major depressive disorder, the dose of TCA should be increased to antidepressant dosage levels. If this is not tolerated, an SSRI may be tried as an alternative. For patients who are especially anxious, alprazolam can be considered. Tramadol (Ultram) was found to produce statistically significant improvement in patient-reported pain scores and pain relief ratings.

For FM, regular exercise is of paramount importance. Research centers that use a multidisciplinary approach to treatment have found that cardiovascular fitness training improves both subjective and objective measurements of pain. Any fitness program must be started at a low level because FM patients are often quite deconditioned and overdoing may exacerbate symptoms. The exercise should be nonimpact loading (e.g., walking or Nordic track). The exercycle is especially good because it avoids stress on tender points in the lower extremities. Extremely deconditioned patients should be started with water aerobics. Exercise sessions should be followed by gentle stretching. Yoga and tai chi are two good activities for patients with FM. Exercise should be done three or four times per week at about 70% maximum heart rate for 20 to 30 minutes at a time. Patients should be cautioned to be patient and should be given lots of encouragement because it may take 3 to 6 months to begin to see a benefit. If classes are not available or patients find the cost prohibitive, instructional videos are available on exercise, yoga, and tai chi.

Other measures that have been found to be beneficial in FM are biofeedback and hypnotherapy. Electromyographic (EMG) biofeedback versus a mock procedure showed improvement in ratings on a visual analog pain scale, morning stiffness, and the number of tender points. Differences remained 5 months after treatment. Hypnotherapy compared with physical therapy showed improvement in visual analog pain ratings, sleep measures, patient's global assessment, and somatic and psychic discomfort scores. This improvement was maintained 6 months after treatment.

The range of treatment options is wide and varied. Patients may be overwhelmed and not know how to choose. Choices can be made based on availability in the community, cost, and patient temperament.

Cognitive behavior therapy (CBT) has been shown to be helpful in patients with FM. It is apparent that there are common beliefs among many FM patients that contribute to the perpetuation of their symptoms. These beliefs include the following:
• They are to blame for the pain.
• The pain is mysterious.
• The pain will continue.

Patients who hold these beliefs have more pain, less adherence to treatment, poorer self-esteem, more somatization, and greater psychic distress.

It is also clear that patients' feelings of self-efficacy (i.e., one's ability to make an impact on one's current situation) are a significant determinant of the affective experience of pain (the emotional upheaval that the unpleasant experience of pain arouses). Patients with high self-efficacy tend to engage in coping behaviors until success is achieved. Those with low self-efficacy more quickly discontinue coping strategies because they anticipate failure.

CBT encourages patients to examine and challenge these negative beliefs and to foster feelings of self-efficacy. Patients look at ways in which they have assumed the sick role and how that interferes with improvement. With CBT, patients examine the role that stress plays in their lives and are supported to find ways to reduce their stress through problem-solving techniques.

Studies using CBT found improved psychiatric outcomes, less distress, less pain, and less interference with regular activities. Follow-up studies showed changes persisting at 2.5 years.

Follow-up

FM is generally a chronic syndrome. Patients should be seen regularly, possibly every 1 to 2 months on first diagnosis. This allows the physician to support patients' efforts at exercise and positive behaviors.

It is often a condition that waxes and wanes, based on stressors in the patient's life. Patients should be encouraged to see their physicians sooner rather than later if they feel their symptoms worsening.

Patient Education

FM is an illness where a supportive relationship with a physician is of paramount importance. Educating patients about FM takes great diplomacy. They should be reassured of the following:

• FM is not life-threatening.
• Their symptoms are not imagined.
• Their pain will not result in joint deformities.
• Although complete remissions are rare, symptoms do appear to improve over time.

Physicians should acknowledge that although a medical explanation for FM has not been forthcoming, the patient's suffering is real. At the same time, physicians must dissuade patients from a belief that extensive diagnostic testing might uncover an occult illness.

Physicians can incorporate some principles of CBT into patient care in the following ways. To evaluate the extent to which the patient has assumed the sick role, ask what activities have been given up. Patients may need to keep an activity log for a few weeks to discern these changes. Patients can be given homework assignments to return to those activities. Helping patients find opportunities for success will improve their self-efficacy and self-esteem. Ask patients to articulate their fears about the long-term effects of their illness so these can be counteracted. Problem-solve with patients about ways to mitigate stress in their lives. Stress the importance of good sleep hygiene: avoidance of caffeine or other stimulants, avoidance of daytime napping, and promotion of the bedroom as a haven that is quiet and free of distractions. Finally, emphasize the importance of regular exercise and helping patients develop a concrete strategy for getting into an exercise program.

CHRONIC FATIGUE SYNDROME

Chronic fatigue syndrome (CFS) shares many similarities with FM. The predominant symptom in CFS is a pervasive, overwhelming fatigue, whereas pain or tenderness is the hallmark of FM. There is considerable comorbidity between CFS and FM.

As with FM, the diagnostic label may be new, but descriptions of CFS date back to the middle of the nineteenth century. At various times this syndrome has been called neurasthenia, benign myalgic encephalomyelitis, or chronic Epstein-Barr virus infection.

Chief Complaint

- A 56-year-old former clerical worker presents with the symptom of fatigue to the extent that she's been unable to work for the past 2 months. At various times she feels as if she's feverish or chilled. Her muscles and joints ache much of the time. The most troubling symptom for her is a feeling of being in a mental "fog."

Clinical Manifestations

The Centers for Disease Control (CDC) convened an expert panel in the late 1980s to develop a working definition of CFS. The panel came up with two major criteria, 11 minor criteria, and three physical examination criteria (Table 10.2).

Other symptoms frequently offered by CFS patients that are not included in the CDC criteria include the following:

- Unusually low basal body temperature
- Soft neurologic signs, such as difficulty with Romberg's testing and tandem gait

T ABLE 10.2.   CDC diagnostic criteria for chronic fatigue syndrome

Both major and either eight minor, or six minor symptoms and at least two physical examination criteria, must be present to fulfill the case definition

I. Major criteria
   A. Persistence of relapsing fatigue or easy fatigability that does not resolve with bed rest and is severe enough to reduce average daily activity by at least 50% for at least 6 months
   B. Other chronic conditions have been satisfactorily excluded, including chronic psychiatric illness*
II. Minor symptom criteria
   A. Mild fever (37.5–38.6°C [99.5–101.4°F] orally) or chills
   B. Sore throat
   C. Posterior cervical, anterior cervical, or axillary lymph node pain
   D. Unexplained generalized muscle weakness
   E. Muscle discomfort or myalgia
   F. Prolonged (at least 24 hours) generalized fatigue following previously tolerable levels of exercise
   G. New, generalized headaches
   H. Migratory, noninflammatory arthralgias
   I. Neuropsychiatric symptoms, photophobia, transient visual scotoma, forgetfulness, excessive irritability, confusion, difficulty thinking, inability to concentrate, depression
   J. Sleep disturbance (hypersomnia or insomnia)
   K. Patient's description of initial onset of symptoms as acute or subacute
III. Physical examination criteria
   Must be documented by a physician on at least two occasions, at least 1 month apart
   A. Low-grade fever (37.6–38.6°C [99.6–101.4°F] orally or 37.8–38.8°C [100.1–101.8°F] rectally)
   B. Nonexudative pharyngitis
   C. Palpable or tender anterior cervical, posterior cervical, or axillary lymph nodes (<2 cm in diameter)

*It is no longer recommended that chronic psychiatric illness be a reason for exclusion.

- Anisocoria (inequality in diameter of the pupils)
- Night sweats

The problems with cognition and sleep are commonly most distressing to patients.

In subsequent years, problems have arisen with using a criteria-based diagnosis. The criteria do not define a unique patient group, and they have not been empirically tested. It has also become clear that physicians do not uniformly apply the criteria. One major problem with the CDC's guidelines was the original exclusion of any patient who had psychiatric comorbidity. The original authors of the guidelines have recommended that this exclusion be eliminated.

Epidemiology

Estimates of the prevalence of CFS are hard to come by because case definition has been difficult. Most people feel fatigue at one time or another. A British study found that 20% of respondents stated that they were tired all the time, but most did not identify it as a medical problem. A group in Australia found the prevalence to be 39.6 cases per 100,000, whereas another group in New Zealand found a much higher prevalence of 127 cases per 100,000.

Of patients diagnosed with CFS, 73% are women, 63% are college graduates, and the average length of fatigue was 7 years. Ninety percent had cut down on social and recreational activities, and more than half were unable to work full-time.

Australian researchers found that patients with CFS had an average of 18 visits per year to their primary care provider and specialists, and an additional 14 visits per year to acupuncturists, physical therapists, chiropractors, and other nonphysician practitioners.

Risk Factors

The most common comorbidities with CFS are the following:
- Major depressive disorder
- Panic disorder
- General anxiety disorder
- Somatization disorder

There are four possible explanations for the concurrence of CFS and psychiatric illness:
- The syndrome is predominantly a psychiatric diagnosis mislabeled as CFS.
- The psychiatric symptoms are secondary to CFS and are the predictable response to having a disabling, poorly understood illness. Alternatively, the symptoms may be organic, based on an as yet poorly understood brain lesion.
- CFS and psychiatric symptoms are both part of an undefined primary illness.
- The primary illness is CFS and the psychiatric diagnosis is wrong.

It is not clear at this time which may be the correct hypothesis, and it is likely that different ones may apply to different patients.

In the past medical history only allergies were found more frequently among patients with CFS than among the general population. Sixty percent to 80% of patients with CFS were found to have a history of allergies or atopic illness.

Pathology

A defining lesion has not been discovered in CFS, although recent research appears to be coalescing in certain areas. The following hypotheses have been explored:
- **Infection.** A total of 10 infectious agents have been investigated as potential causes of CFS (Table 10.3). None of the preceding qualifies as the sole causative agent for CFS, but it appears that several may act along with other cofactors to produce CFS.

T ABLE 10.3. Infectious agents investigated as possible causes of chronic fatigue syndrome

Brucella
Influenza
Enteroviruses (including Coxsackieviruses)
Epstein-Barr virus
Candida
Human herpesvirus type 6
Retroviruses
Borrelia burgdorferii

- **Immunologic dysfunction.** Abnormalities have been found in virtually every aspect of lymphoid functioning, yet it is difficult to know what to make of the findings. They are not found in every patient, and in most cases do not represent a sharp deviation from normal. It is also not understood whether the immune findings are primary or secondary.
- **Muscle tissue.** When muscle tissue, metabolism, and physiology have been examined, no consistent findings have been found that explain CFS on the basis of a muscular disease.
- **Neuroendocrine function.** Studies examining levels of neuroendocrine hormones have found a reduction in the output of adrenal glucocorticoids. It is postulated that there is a CNS-mediated failure in the activation of the hypothalamic pituitary adrenal (HPA) axis.

Diagnosis

Table 10.4 lists the differential diagnosis for CFS. A reasonable laboratory evaluation to evaluate fatigue would include the following:
- Complete blood count
- Manual differential looking for the presence of atypical lymphocytes
- Sedimentation rate
- Chemistry panel, including renal and liver function tests, glucose, electrolytes, calcium, phosphate, cholesterol, albumin, and globulin levels
- TSH levels
- Antinuclear antibodies and rheumatoid factor (if arthralgias are prominent)
- Urinalysis

Centers that specialize in the diagnosis and treatment of CFS typically do an indepth analysis of multiple immune parameters, but these are generally not available to the practicing physician and have not been proved to have reasonable specificity and sensitivity.

Magnetic resonance imaging (MRI) in patients with CFS has occasionally shown hyperintensities, but these findings are inconsistent. At this point, it does not appear that MRI is a useful diagnostic procedure for CFS.

Referral

Whether a physician wants to undertake the care of patients with CFS depends on his or her inclination and the availability of someone else in the community with that interest. There are centers and physicians who devote much of their practice to the care of patients with CFS, but they are not widely available, nor has there been

T ABLE 10.1. Differential diagnosis of CFS—conditions with an initial presentation of fatigue but that do not meet CDC criteria for CFS

Psychiatric illness
  Major depressive disorder
  Generalized anxiety disorder
  Somatization disorder
  Panic disorder
Endocrinopathies
  Hypothyroidism
  Hyperthyroidism
  Diabetes mellitus
Multiple sclerosis
Collagen vascular disease
  Systemic lupus erythematosus
Renal failure
Hepatitis
Sleep disturbance
  Nocturnal myoclonus
  Narcolepsy

Abbreviation: CFS, chronic fatigue syndrome.

research showing that this kind of care improves patient outcomes. A sympathetic physician with a willing ear and the ability to coordinate care among ancillary services can be of great assistance to these patients.

Management

No single accepted treatment exists for CFS. However, many things have been tried and appear successful in some patients. The first task is to assess for the presence of an Axis I diagnosis. If such a disorder is present, it should be treated with the appropriate pharmacotherapy. If no Axis I diagnosis exists, troublesome symptoms should be targeted and treated symptomatically.

Other treatments that have been tried experimentally include the following. Intravenous IgG was found to improve symptoms in one study, but relief was transient. One study, reported in *Lancet,* showed the use of low-dose hydrocortisone (5 to 40 mg per day) reduced self-reports of fatigue and disability. Others have treated presumed hypoadrenalism with dehydroepiandrosterone (DHEA). Ampligen, a mixture of double-stranded DNA, is undergoing research trials after anecdotal reports showed effectiveness. Anecdotal reports credit symptom improvement to a combination of methylphenidate and phentermine. One randomized controlled clinical trial showed improvement in symptom scores over placebo when patients were given high-dose essential fatty acids. Nefazodone (Serzone) was found in one small study to improve fatigue, sleep, and mood when compared with placebo.

Other methods that have been found to be helpful with CFS include the following:
- **A program of gradually increasing activity.** This should be started at a low level, and patients should be instructed to attempt to achieve 60% of maximal heart rate based on age. From their daily experiences, patients have learned that exertion is frequently followed by exacerbations of their fatigue and are understandably

reluctant to try exercise. One approach that appears helpful is to rotate 4 to 8 minutes of exercise with 4 minutes of rest. This can be done in three or four cycles.
- **Extra salt and water intake.** It has recently been recognized that many patients with CFS also have neurally mediated hypotension. If symptoms suggest orthostasis, patients can be tested using a tilt table or simple office orthostatics. Having the patient drink lots of water during the day and take extra salt may alleviate these symptoms.
- **Cognitive behavior therapy (CBT).** This has also been found to be helpful in CFS. CBT addresses modifiable lifestyle factors that contribute to the patient's fear of disability. Through CBT, patients examine the extent to which they have assumed the sick role and the role that stress is playing in their illness. Patients are instructed to look at their beliefs about meeting others' expectations and their own need to perform to perfectionist standards.

Follow-up

Patients with CFS should be seen on a regular basis so that the physician can provide support for lifestyle changes and be aware of exacerbations. Patients can be given homework to do between visits, such as keeping a diary of exercise or daily activities, trying new activities, attempting stress reduction techniques, or being more assertive.

Patient Education

Once again, it is crucial for physicians to forge a therapeutic alliance with CFS patients so that they feel they are being heard. Physicians must stress that they believe that the patient is suffering, even though there is no currently understood cause for this illness. At the same time, the physician must help the patient identify behaviors and beliefs that interfere with the patient's getting better. Negative beliefs about the consequences of exercise and a strong belief that one is suffering from an as yet undiagnosed medical illness were two predictors of poor outcome and greater disability.

SUGGESTED READINGS

Ang D, Wilke WS. Diagnosis, etiology and therapy of fibromyalgia. *Compr Ther* 1999; 25:221.

Barsky AJ, Borus JF. Functional somatic syndromes. *Ann Intern Med* 1999;130:910.

Bennett RM. Emerging concepts in the neurobiology of chronic pain: evidence of abnormal sensory processing in fibromyalgia. *Mayo Clin Proc* 1999;74:385.

Clear AJ, Heap E, Malhi GD, et al. Low-dose hydrocortisone in chronic fatigue syndrome: a randomized cross-over trial. *Lancet* 1999;353:455.

Dawson DM, Sabin TD. *Chronic fatigue syndrome.* Boston: Little, Brown, 1993.

Hickie I. Nefazodone for patients with chronic fatigue syndrome. *Aust N Z J Psychiatry* 1999;33:278.

Koopman WJ. *Arthritis and allied conditions: a textbook of rheumatology,* vol. 2. Baltimore: Williams & Wilkins, 1997.

Leventhal LJ. Management of fibromyalgia. *Ann Intern Med* 1999;131:850.

Moldofsky H, Scarisbrick P, England R, et al. Musculoskeletal symptoms and non-REM sleep disturbances in patients with "fibrositis" syndrome and healthy subjects. *Psychosom Med* 1975:37:341.

Sharpe M. Cognitive behavior therapy for chronic fatigue syndrome: efficacy and implications. *Am J Med* 1998;105:104S.

Straus SE. *Chronic fatigue syndrome.* New York: Marcel Dekker, 1994.

SUBJECT INDEX

References in italics indicate figures; those followed by "t" denote tables

A

Abstinence, 11, *13*
Adolescents, contraceptive methods for, 25-26
Alprazolam, 116
Amenorrhea, 19t
Amitriptyline, 115t
Amoxapine, 115t
Angina
   description of, 73
   treatment, 82, 82t
Antidepressants. *See* Heterocyclic
      antidepressants; Monoamine oxidase
      inhibitors; Selective serotonin reuptake
      inhibitors; Tricyclic antidepressants
Arthritis. *See* Osteoarthritis; Rheumatoid arthritis
Asendin. *See* Amoxapine
Aspirin, 78, 82t
Atypical squamous cells of undetermined
      significance (ASCUS), 33

B

BCa. *See* Breast cancer
Beta-blockers, 82t
Binge-eating disorder
   chief complaint, 95
   clinical manifestations of, 95
   definition of, 95
   diagnosis of, 96, 96t
   epidemiology of, 95
   follow-up, 97
   management of, 97
   patient education, 97
   referral, 96
   risk factors, 95-96
Biopsy
   open surgical, 52
   stereotactic-guided breast, 52
Biphosphonates, for osteoporosis, 144
Body mass index
   coronary heart disease risk and, 75, *76*
   health risks and, *88*
   obesity classifications and, 87
   osteoarthritis risks and, 136
BRCA1, 56-57
BRCA2, 56-57
Breakthrough bleeding
   description of, 18t, 19
   treatment, 23t
Breast cancer (BCa). *See* Cancer
Breast cysts, 46-47
Breast disease, 6t
Breastfeeding, contraceptive use during, 26, 26t
Breast mass
   description of, 46-47
   referral indications, 52t, 53

Bulimia nervosa
   behaviors associated with, 95
   chief complaint, 95
   clinical manifestations of, 95
   definition of, 95
   diagnosis of, 96, 96t
   epidemiology of, 95
   follow-up, 97
   management of, 96-97
   patient education, 97
   referral, 96
   risk factors, 95-96
Bupropion, 115t, 126

C

Calcitonin, for osteoporosis, 144
Calcium channel blockers, for angina, 82t
Cancer
   breast (BCa)
      age-based incidence of, 47, *49*
      axillary nodal involvement, 55
      chief complaints, 45
      clinical manifestations of
         cysts, 46-47
         lumps, 46
         masses, 46-47
         nipple discharge, 45t, 45-46, *46*
         pain, 45
         vague nodularity, 47
      contraception methods and, 10-11
      diagnostic and evaluative approach
         biopsies, 52
         Doppler sonography, 52
         examination, 51
         fine-needle aspiration, 52
         mammography, 51, 51t
         stereotactic-guided breast biopsy, 52
         ultrasound, 51
      epidemiology of, 47
      estrogen replacement therapy and, 66
      genetic indicators, 56-57
      prognostic factors, 56, 57t
      recurrence rates, 56
      risk factors, 48-49
      screening, 49-51
      staging of, 53, 55-56
      survival rates, 55t, 56
      treatment
         chemotherapy, 56
         mastectomy, 53, 57
         radiation, 53, 54t, 56
         stage-based, 53-56, 54t
         surgery, 53, 54t
   cervical
      chief complaint, 29

Cancer (*contd*)
 clinical manifestations of, 29
 diagnostic and evaluative approach
  colposcopy, 33, *34*
  Pap smear, 31-33
 epidemiology of, 29, *30*
 ethnic predilection, 29, *30*
 follow-up, 37
 management of, 33-36
 pathology, 31
 referral, 34
 risk factors, 30-31
 staging of, 36t
 survival rates, 36, *36*
 endometrial
  chief complaint, 37
  clinical manifestations of, 37
  diagnosis of, *39*, 38
  epidemiology of, 37
  estrogen replacement therapy and, 38, 65t
  follow-up, 39
  management of, 38
  pathology, 38
  risk factors, 37t, 37-38
  staging of, 38, 40t
  survival rates, 39, 40t
 ovarian
  chief complaint, 40
  clinical manifestations of, 40
  diagnosis of, 41, *41-42*
  epidemiology of, 40
  follow-up, 43
  prophylactic oophorectomy for, 57
  risk factors, 41
  screening tests for, 42
Carcinoembryonic antigen, for ovarian cancer
  screening, 42
Celexa. *See* Citalopram
Cervical cancer. *See* Cancer
Cervical cap, 10, 15-16
CFS. *See* Chronic fatigue syndrome
CHD. *See* Coronary heart disease
Chronic fatigue syndrome (CFS)
 chief complaint, 152
 clinical manifestations of, 152-153
 description of, 151
 diagnosis of, 152t, 154, 155t
 differential diagnosis, 154, 155t
 epidemiology of, 153
 follow-up, 156
 management of, 155-156
 pathology associated with, 153-154, 154t
 patient education, 156
 referral, 154
 risk factors, 153
Cigarette smoking. *See* Smoking
Citalopram, 115t
Cognitive behavior therapy
 for chronic fatigue syndrome, 156
 for fibromyalgia, 150-151
Coitus interruptus, 5, 7, 11-12
Colposcopy, for cervical cancer evaluations, 33,
  34

Condoms, *13*, 14-15
Contraception
 for adolescents, 25-26
 for breastfeeding women, 26, 26t
 cancer concerns, 10-11
 considerations before initiating
  abnormal Pap tests, 4
  availability, 5, 7
  costs, 5, 9t
  future fertility decisions, 2, 2t
  gynecologic abnormalities, 4
  medication use, 5, 8t
  menstrual disorders, 2, 4
  occupation, 8-9, 9t
  orderliness of life, 8
  preexisting medical conditions, 4t 7t,
   4-5
  sexual experiences, 7
 for disabled women, 27t, 27-28
 emergency, 16-17
 methods
  abstinence, 11, 13
  barrier, 14-16
  cervical cap, 10, 15-16
  coitus interruptus, 5, 7, 11-12
  concerns regarding, 10-11
  condoms, *13*, 14-15
  creams, 14
  Depo-Provera, 21, 21t 22t
  diaphragm, *13*, 15
  gels, 14
  hormonal. *See* Oral contraceptives
  implantable, 22t 23t, 22-23
  injectable, 21, 21t 22t
  IUDs, 23-24
  natural family planning, 13-14
  oral contraceptive pills (OCP). *See* Oral
   contraceptives
  overview of, 1t
  rhythm, 12-13
  spermicides, *13*, 14
  sterilization, *13*, 24
  suppositories, 14
 for older women, 26-27
 reversibility considerations, 2
 side effects, 10, *10*
Coronary artery bypass grafting, 83
Coronary heart disease (CHD)
 angina associated with, 73
 cardiac catheterization evaluations, 81-82
 chief complaint, 73
 clinical manifestations of, 73-74
 description of, 73
 diagnostic and evaluative approach, 80-81, *81*
 epidemiology of, 74
 prevention of
  primary, 78, 79t
  secondary, 78-80, 79t
 referrals, 81-82
 risk factors
  body mass index, 75, *76*
  diabetes mellitus, 77
  employment, 75

family history, 75
gender, 74
hypertension, 77
lifestyle, 77
lipid levels, 77
menopause, 77-78
obesity, 75
oral contraceptives, 77
psychosocial factors, 74, 75, *76*
race, 74, *74*, 75t
smoking, 75, 77
stratification of, 78-80, 79t
treatment of
coronary artery bypass grafting, 83
medical, 82, 82t
percutaneous transluminal coronary
angioplasty, 82-83
surgical, 82-83
Cryosurgery, for cervical dysplasia, 35
Cysts, breast, 46-47

D
Deep venous thrombosis
estrogen replacement therapy and, 65t
oral contraceptive use and, 11
Depomedroxyprogesterone/Depo-Provera, 21,
21t 22t
Depression. *See also* Premenstrual dysphoric
disorder
in bulimia nervosa patient, 95
chief complaint, 103
clinical manifestations of, 103t, 103-104
definition of, 103
diagnosis of, 105-106
drugs associated with, 105t
epidemiology of, 104
female-specific assessment of, 106t
follow-up, 109-110
management of
algorithms, *111-113*
electroconvulsive therapy, 108
exercise, 109
light therapy, 109
medications, 106-108, 110, 115t. *See also*
specific medication
psychotherapy, 107-108
St. John's wort, 109
medical conditions associated with, 105t
menopause and, 60
oral contraceptive use and, 6t, 18t
pathology of, 104
patient education, 113-114
postpartum. *See* Postpartum depression
referral, 106
risk factors, 104
suicide risks, 110, 112
symptoms of, 103t
Desipramine, 115t
Desyrel. *See* Trazodone
Diabetes mellitus
coronary heart disease risk and, 77
oral contraceptive use, 6t
Diaphragm, *13*, 15

Disabled women, contraception for, 27t, 27-28
Doxepin, 115t
Dysmenorrhea, 2, 4
Dyspareunia
chief complaint, 127-128
clinical manifestations of, 128
definition of, 127
diagnosis of, 129-130
epidemiology of, 128
follow-up, 130-131
management of, 130
pathology associated with, 129
patient education regarding, 131
referral, 130
risk factors, 128-129
secondary, 129, 129t
Dysthymia, 104

E
Eating disorders. *See* Binge-eating disorder;
Bulimia nervosa
Effexor. *See* Venlafaxine
Elavil. *See* Amitriptyline
Electroconvulsive therapy, 108
Emergency contraception, 16-17
Endometrial cancer. *See* Cancer
Estrogen replacement therapy
algorithm for assessing need, *63*
breast cancer and, 66
compliance with, 66
complications associated with, 66
conditions benefited by, 62t
considerations before initiating, 66, 68t 69t
contraindications, 65t, 66
coronary heart disease risk and, 78
description of, 61
endometrial cancer and, 38, 65t
estrogen-progestin combinations, 64t, 65
estrogens, 62
fractures and, *142*, 142-143
monitoring of, 66
osteoarthritis and, 136
products, 68t 69t
progestin, 62-63
regimen, 63-65, 64t
Exercise
for chronic fatigue syndrome, 155
for depression, 109
for fibromyalgia, 150
for obesity, 90

F
Fibromyalgia (FM)
chief complaint, 145
clinical manifestations of, 145-147, *146*
definition of, 145
diagnosis of, 148, 149t
epidemiology of, 147
follow-up, 151
management of
cognitive behavior therapy, 150-151
medications, 149-150
pathology associated with, 148

Fibromyalgia (FM) (*contd*)
  patient education, 151
  referral, 149
  risk factors, 147
Fine-needle aspiration, for breast cancer
  diagnosis, 52
Fluoxetine, 115t
FM. *See* Fibromyalgia
Food groups
  glycemic index, 99t
  serving sizes, 90t 91t

G
Gallbladder disease, 6t
Gestational diabetes, 6t
Gonadotrophin-releasing hormone, 116
Gynecologic cancer. *See* specific cancer

H
Heart disease. *See* Coronary heart disease
Hepatic disease, 6t
Heterocyclic antidepressants, 115t
Hormone replacement therapy. *See* Estrogen
  replacement therapy
Hot flashes, 59, 67
HSDD. *See* Hypoactive sexual desire disorder
Human papillomavirus, cervical cancer and,
  30
Hyperlipidemia
  coronary heart disease risk and, 77
  oral contraceptives use, 6t
Hypertension
  coronary heart disease risk and, 77
  oral contraceptive use, 6t
Hypoactive sexual desire disorder (HSDD)
  chief complaint, 123
  clinical manifestations of, 123
  description of, 122-123
  diagnosis of, 124
  drugs associated with, 125t
  epidemiology of, 123
  follow-up, 126-127
  management of, 126, 127t
  patient education, 127
  referral, 124-126
  risk factors, 123-124, 124t

I
Imipramine, 115t
Intrauterine devices (IUDs), 23-24
Isocarboxazid, 115t

K
Kegel exercises, 133

L
Levonorgestrel, 3t, 22t-23t, 22-23, 64t
Lipids
  coronary heart disease risk and, 77
  elevated levels of. *See* Hyperlipidemia
Loop electrosurgical excision procedure, for
  cervical dysplasia, 35, 35t
Ludiomil. *See* Maprotiline

M
Magnetic resonance imaging
  for breast cancer screening and staging, 50, 53
  for rheumatoid arthritis evaluation, 139
Mammography, for breast cancer evaluation,
  49-51, 51t
MAOIs. *See* Monoamine oxidase inhibitors
Maprotiline, 115t
Marplan. *See* Isocarboxazid
Menopause
  chief complaint, 59
  clinical manifestations of, 59-60
  coronary heart disease risk and, 77-78
  description of, 59
  diagnosis of, 61
  epidemiology of, 60
  estrogen replacement therapy. See Estrogen
    replacement therapy
  pathology of, 60-61
  patient education, 67, 70
  referral, 61
  risk factors, 60
  treatment of
    alternative, 66-67
    estrogen replacement therapy. *See* Estrogen
      replacement therapy
    lifestyle changes, 67
Menorrhagia
  IUD use and, 24
  oral contraceptive use and, 2, 4, 19t
  treatment for, 23t
Menstruation
  cessation of. *See* Menopause
  disorders of, 2, 4, 19t, 23t. *See also* specific
    disorder
Metabolic syndrome
  chief complaint, 97
  clinical manifestations of, 97-98
  description of, 97
  diagnosis of, 98-99
  epidemiology of, 98
  follow-up, 100
  management of, 99-100
  pathology associated with, 98
  patient education regarding, 100
  referral, 99
  risk factors, 98
Mifepristone, 16t
Migraine headaches
  estrogen replacement therapy and, 65t
  oral contraceptive use and, 6t
Mitral valve prolapse, 7t
Monoamine oxidase inhibitors, 115t
Morning-after pill, 16-17
MRI. *See* Magnetic resonance imaging

N
Nardil. *See* Phenelzine
Natural family planning, 13-14
Nipple discharge, 45t, 45-46, *46*
Nitrates, for angina, 82t
Nonsteroidal anti-inflammatory drugs (NSAIDS)
  complications associated with, 138, 138t

for osteoarthritis, 138
Norgestrel, 3t, 19
Norplant, 22t 23t, 22-23
Norpramin. *See* Desipramine
Norethindrone, 3t, 19, 64t
Nortriptyline, 115t
NSAIDs. *See* Nonsteroidal anti-inflammatory
    drugs

O
Obesity
    chief complaint, 85
    clinical manifestations of, 85-86
    coronary heart disease risk and, 75
    description of, 85
    diagnosis of, 87
    epidemiology of, 86
    follow-up, 93
    management of
        behavioral approach, 90-91
        calorie counting, 89-90
        exercise, 90
        medications, 91, 92t
        overview of, 88-89
        surgical, 91-93, 92t
        weight loss, 89t, 89-90, 93-94
    oral contraceptive use, 7t
    pathology of, 87
    patient education, 93-94
    referral, 87
    risk factors, 86-87
OCPs. *See* Oral contraceptives
Older women, contraception for, 26-27
Oligomenorrhea, 4, 19t
Oral contraceptives. *See also* Contraception
    breakthrough bleeding secondary to, 18t, 19
    combination, 17-18
    concerns regarding
        cancer, 10-11, 17t
        coronary heart disease, 77
        deep venous thrombosis, 11
    contraindications, 4t 5t
    costs of, 9t
    Depo-Provera, 21, 21t 22t
    endometrial activity associated with, 20t
    medications that affect, 8t
    noncontraceptive benefits of, 17t
    Norplant, 22t 23t, 22-23
    osteoporosis and, 143
    progestational activity associated with, 20t
    progestin-only, 19, 21
    rheumatoid arthritis and, 139
    side effects, 17-19, 18t 20t
    types of, 1t, 3t
Orgasmic disorders, 131-133
Osteoarthritis
    chief complaint, 135
    clinical manifestations of, 135
    description of, 135
    diagnosis of, 136-137
    differential diagnosis, 137t
    epidemiology of, 135
    estrogen replacement therapy and, 136

follow-up, 139
    management of, 138
    referral, 138-139
    risk factors, 135-136, *136*
Osteoporosis
    chief complaints, 140
    clinical manifestations of, 140
    definition of, 140
    diagnosis of, 143
    epidemiology of, 140
    follow-up, 144
    hip fractures secondary to, 141, 142t
    management of, 143-144
    menopause and, 60
    oral contraceptive use and, 11
    prevention of
        calcium supplementation, 143
        estrogen replacement therapy, *142*,
            142-143
        oral contraceptives use, 143
        overview of, 141-142
        vitamin D supplementation, 143
    risk factors, 140-141, 141t
Ovarian cancer. *See* Cancer

P
Pamelor. *See* Nortriptyline
Pap smear
    cervical cancer diagnosis, 31-33
    contraception and, 4
    evaluative algorithm, *32*
    indications, 31
Parnate. *See* Tranylcypromine
Paroxetine (Paxil), 115t
Percutaneous transluminal coronary angioplasty,
    82-83
Periodic abstinence, 12-13
Phenelzine, 115t
Pill. *See* Oral contraceptives
Plan B, 16
Postpartum depression
    chief complaint, 116
    clinical manifestations of, 117
    diagnosis of, 117-118
    epidemiology of, 117
    management of, 118
    pathology associated with, 117
    patient education, 118
    referral, 118
    risk factors, 117
Premenstrual dysphoric disorder. *See also*
        Depression
    chief complaint, 114
    clinical manifestations of, 114, 115t
    diagnosis of, 115
    epidemiology of, 114
    follow-up, 116
    management of, 115-116
    pathology associated with, 114
    patient education, 116
    referral, 115
    risk factors, 114
Preven, 16

Progesterone, 62
Progestin
  contraceptive uses of
    injectable, 21, 21t 23t
    oral contraceptive, 19, 21
  estrogen replacement therapy use, 62–63, 64t
Protriptyline, 115t
Prozac. *See* Fluoxetine
PTCA. *See* Percutaneous transluminal coronary
  angioplasty

R
Rheumatoid arthritis, 139–140
Rhythm method, 12–13
Roux-en-y gastric bypass, for obesity
  management, 92t
RU-486. *See* Mifepristone

S
Seizure disorders, 7t
Selective serotonin reuptake inhibitors (SSRIs).
  See also specific drug
  for depression, 115t
  for fibromyalgia, 149–150
  side effects, 115t
  types of, 115t
Sertraline, 115t
Sexual problems
  drugs associated with, 125t
  dyspareunia. *See* Dyspareunia
  history-taking regarding, 121t 122t
  hypoactive sexual desire disorder. *See*
    Hypoactive sexual desire disorder
  orgasmic disorders, 131–133
  overview of, 121
Sickle cell disease, 7t
Sinequan. *See* Doxepin
Smoking
  cervical cancer and, 31
  coronary heart disease risk and, 75, 77
  estrogen replacement therapy and,
    65t
  menopause onset and, 60
Spermicides, 13, 14
SSRIs. *See* Selective serotonin reuptake
  inhibitors
Stereotactic-guided breast biopsy, for breast
  cancer diagnosis, 52
Sterilization, 24
Stroke
  estrogen replacement therapy and, 65t
  oral contraceptive use and, 11
Suicide, 110, 112
Surmontil. *See* Trimipramine
Syndrome X. *See* Metabolic syndrome
Systemic lupus erythematosus

estrogen replacement therapy and, 65t
oral contraceptive use and, 7t

T
Tamoxifen
  for breast cancer, 56
  endometrial cancer and, 38
TCA. *See* Tricyclic antidepressants
Thrombosis. *See* Deep venous thrombosis
Tobacco use. *See* Smoking
Tofranil. *See* Imipramine
Tranylcypromine, 115t
Trazodone, 115t, 126
Tricyclic antidepressants. *See also*
    specific drug
  for depression, 115t
  for fibromyalgia, 149–150
  side effects, 115t
  types of, 115t
Trimipramine, 115t
Tubal ligation, *13*, 24

U
Ulcerative colitis, 7t
Ultrasound
  for breast cancer diagnosis, 51
  for ovarian cancer screening, 42

V
Vaginismus, 129
Valvular heart disease, 6t
Vasectomy, 13, 24
Venlafaxine, 115t
Venous thrombosis. *See* Deep venous
  thrombosis
Vertical plastic binding technique, for obesity
  management, 92t
Vivactil. *See* Protriptyline
Vulvar vestibulitis, 128, 1309t
Vulvodynia
  clinical manifestations of, 127–128
  diagnosis of, 130
  management of, 130t
Vulvovaginitis, 128, 130t

W
Weight loss
  for metabolic syndrome, 99
  for obesity management, 89t, 89–90, 93–94
Weight-related issues. *See* Binge-eating
    disorder; Bulimia; Metabolic syndrome;
    Obesity
Wellbutrin. *See* Bupropion

Z
Zoloft. *See* Sertraline

LIPPINCOTT WILLIAMS & WILKINS
Survey for the
American Academy of Family Physicians
Academy Collection

As a purchaser of the *AAFP's Academy Collection,* you are better qualified than anyone else to assess the day-to-day value of these books.
Your perspective would help us plan additional books in the series.

(Please Print)

Name _____

Address_____

City/State/Zip_____

Phone_____Fax _____

E-mail _____

UTILITY OF CONTENT

How are you using the *Academy Collection* titles? In what circumstances do you consult one of the titles in the *Academy Collection*?

What do you like best about this product?

What do you like least about this product?

Consider the content of the books you have purchased from the *Academy Collection*, can you obtain this information from other books/journals?
　❑ Yes (If yes, please list the other publications that you use)
　❑ No

What would you change in upcoming titles in the *Academy Collection*?

What other topics would you like to see covered in the *Academy Collection*?

Academy Collection Survey

American Academy of Family Physicians

Academy Collection Survey

GENERAL

How did you learn about the *Academy Collection*?
- ❏ Advertisement in journal
- ❏ Convention
- ❏ Direct Mail
- ❏ Web
- ❏ Colleague
- ❏ Other:_____

Where/how did you purchase the *Academy Collection*?
- ❏ At a convention
- ❏ Via mail
- ❏ Via fax
- ❏ Via Web
- ❏ Via phone

How do you feel about the price of the *Academy Collection* titles?
- ❏ Very reasonable
- ❏ Reasonable
- ❏ Price seems high compared to other medical products
- ❏ Value outweighs price

Are you a member of the *American Academy of Family Physicians*?
- ❏ Yes
- ❏ No

What other medical books or journals have you purchased in the last 12 months.

_____

_____

Mail your reply to: Lippincott Williams & Wilkins
Att: Jason Rodriguez
530 Walnut Street
Philadelphia, PA 19106-3621

Or fax your reply to: Fax: 1-215-521-8487

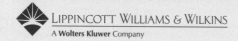

D0A060ZZ